AF658575

DM PULMONARY MEDICINE

ENTRANCE EXAMINATION

(Includes Important Text, Original solved MCQ's and their Explanations)

Editor :

Dr. M.S. Bhatia (M.D.; MNAMS)
Prof & Head, Department of Psychiatry
University College of Medical Sciences &
Guru Teg Bahadur Hospital,
Dilshad Garden Delhi - 110095,

Contributing Editor :

Dr. (Mrs.) Nirmaljit Kaur (M.D.)
Senior Specialist, Department of Microbiology
Dr. R.M.L., Hospital
New Delhi - 110001

CBS

CBS Publishers & Distributors Pvt. Ltd.

New Delhi • Bengaluru • Chennai • Kochi • Kolkata • Mumbai
Hyderabad • Nagpur • Patna • Pune • Vijayawada

Dedicated to
Our Parents and Beloved Children

ISBN: 81-239-1355-9

First Edition: 2006
Reprint: 2007, 2011, 2016, 2019

Copyright © Authors & Publisher

All rights reserved. No part of this book may be reproduced or transmitted in any form or by any means, electronic or mechanical, including photocopying, recording, or any information storage and retrieval system without permission, in writing, from the publisher.

Published by **Satish Kumar Jain** and produced by **Varun Jain** for
CBS Publishers & Distributors Pvt. Ltd.,
4819/XI Prahlad Street, 24 Ansari Road, Daryaganj, New Delhi - 110002
delhi@cbspd.com, cbspubs@airtelmail.in • www.cbspd.com
Ph.: 23289259, 23266861, 23266867 • Fax: 011-23243014

Corporate Office: 204 FIE, Industrial Area, Patparganj, Delhi - 110 092
Ph: 49344934 • Fax: 011-49344935
E-mail: publishing@cbspd.com • publicity@cbspd.com

Branches:
- ***Bengaluru:*** 2975, 17th Cross, K.R. Road, Bansankari 2nd Stage, Bengaluru - 70 • Ph: +91-80-26771678/79 • Fax: +91-80-26771680 E-mail: cbsbng@gmail.com, bangalore@cbspd.com
- ***Chennai:*** No. 7, Subbaraya Street, Shenoy Nagar, Chennai - 600030 Ph: +91-44-26681266, 26680620 • Fax: +91-44-42032115 E-mail: chennai@cbspd.com
- ***Kochi:*** Ashana House, 39/1904, A.M. Thomas Road, Valanjambalam, Ernakulum, Kochi • Ph: +91-484-4059061-65 Fax: +91-484-4059065 • E-mail: cochin@cbspd.com
- ***Kolkata:*** 6-B, Ground Floor, Rameshwar Shaw Road, Kolkata - 700014 Ph: +91-33-22891126/7/8 • E-mail: kolkata@cbspd.com
- ***Mumbai:*** 83-C, Dr. E. Moses Road, Worli, Mumbai - 400018 Ph: +91-9833017933, 022-24902340/41 • E-mail: mumbai@cbspd.com

Representatives:
- Hyderabad: 0-9885175004
- Patna: 0-9334159340
- Jharkhand: 0-9811541605
- Nagpur: 0-9021734563
- Pune: 0-9623451994
- Uttarakhand: 0-9716462459

Printed at: J.S. Offset Printers, Delhi (India)

PREFACE

Medical science is a rapidly advancing field. Its new allied branches are coming up. In a competitive examination, more and more emphasis is being laid on these allied disciplines. But most of the standard textbooks of medicine have failed to devote adequate space to these new disciplines.

This book has been written with the aim to outline the major areas of Pulmonary Medicine i.e Factual data, Commonest symptoms or cause, Named signs and syndromes and *Recent advances.* This book is not merely an addition to the existing list of books on MCQ's but a sincere ambition and an honest attempt to make it a useful and practical companion to both medical graduates and postgraduates. The present book consists of original solved MCQ's from the *Question Banks* of various important examinations (AIIMS, Delhi, PGI etc.), Important text, original solved MCQ's and their explanations have been added. We hope that this will help the candidates in performing better in the examination.

All suggestions for the modification of this book are welcome and will be duly acknowledged.

—Editors

CONTENTS

IMPORTANT TEXT OF PULMONARY MEDICINE

IMPORTANT POINTS TO REMEMBER

* Peak expiratory flow rate is **4-5 X Max. Breathing Capacity (120-150 L/min)** – 500-600 L/min. It is important in COAD (and not in Restrictive disease).
* Signs and symptoms of consolidation in lober pneumonia appear in **2 days** whereas X-ray findings after **12-18 hours.**
* Total lung capacity in male is approx **6.0 L/min** whereas in female it is **4.2 L/min.**
* FEV_1 is **83%** after 1 sec. and **97%** in 3 secs.
* Dead air space is about **150 ml.**
* Massive hemoptysis: **200-600 ml/24 hour** or respiratory distress, anemia, or hypotension.
* Complicated parapneumonic effusions, defined by pH ≤ **8.00-7.20,** glucose ≤ **40 mg/dl,** and/or LDH ≥ 1000 IU/ml, require treatment as for empyema.
* Small pulmonary arteries between **40 and 300 microns** exhibit muscular hypertrophy and intimal hyperplasia in PAH.
* A normal perfusion lung scan rules out pulmonary embolism. The chest x-ray may be normal about **10%** of the time.

COMMONEST IN MEDICINE

* **Commonest** type of dyspnoea in cardiac disease - *Exertional dyspnoea.*
* **Commonest** cause of chronic constrictive pericarditis - *Tuberculosis*
* **Commonest** cause of chronic cor pulmonale - *Chronic asthmatic bronchitis.*
* **Commonest** symptom of respiratory disease is *Cough.*
* **Commonest** cause of acute tracheo*bronchitis is viral infection*
* **Commonest** offender in silicosis is *free silica (silicon dioxide).*
* **Commonest** complaint of silicosis is *dyspnea on exertion.*
* **Commonest** involved organ in Boeck's sarcoid is *lungs*
* **Commonest** cause of death in pneumococcal pneumonia is *Shock and pulm. oedema*

* **Commonest** debilitating resp. disease (in VSA) is *chronic bronchitis.*
* **Commonest** cause of chronic bronchitis is *cigarette smoking.*
* **Commonest** cause of atelectasis is *post op. period following major abdominal or thoracic surgery.*
* **Commonest** symptom of all forms of pulmonary *emboli is sudden onset of dyspnea.*
* **Commonest** cause of hydrothorax is *congestive heart failure.*
* **Commonest** cause of haemothorax is *trauma.*
* **Common** aerobic bacteria causing empyema-*coagulase +ve Staphylococcus aureus and gram -ve bacilli*
* **Commonest** anaerobic organisms encountered in empyema - *bacteroides and peptostreptococci.*
* **Commonest** spontaneous pneumothorax - *unknown*
* **Commonest** chronic mediastinitis - *Histoplasmosis, tuberculosis and sarcoidosis* (in that order)
* **Commonest** metastatic lung lesions - *Staphylococcus*
* **Commonest** bronchiolitis in children - *Resp. syncytial virus.*
* **Commonest** viral penumonia in adults - *Influenza*
* **Commonest** viral pneumonia in children - *resp. syncytial virus*
* **Commonest** fungus ball in lung cavity - *Aspergillosis*
* **Commonest** thin walled cavity with pus - *Coccidioidomycosis*
* **Commonest** multiple cavities in lung - *Blastomycosis*
* **Commonest** pulmonary alveolar proteinosis - *Nocardia*
* **Commonest** involvement of chest wall - *Actinomycosis*
* **Commonest** tropical hemoptysis - *paragonimiasis westermani*
* **Commonest** virus producing resolution in asthma - *Measles.*
* **Commonest** pulmonary infiltrations with eosinophilia - *Aspergillosis.*
* Bronchiolitis of early childhood is most often caused by **Resp. Syncytial virus.**
* **Meliodosis** or **Glanders** result due to Pseudomonas infection.
* Treatment of nocardiasis is dapsone (or cotrimoxazole), maduramycosis — Rifampicin (or cotrimoxazole) and actinomycosis — Penicillin.
* Bronchial adenoma may produce carcinoid syndrome, oat cell may secrete ACTH and adenocarcinoma lung is most frequent in young females and may show **Psammoma bodies.**
* Haemoptysis with renal involvement is seen in **Good Pasture's syndrome.**
* Pneumocytis carinii causes pneumonia

* Cough is a side-effect of **Lisinopril** and **enalapril**
* Sarcoidosis may be characterized by paratracheal lymphadenopathy, cardiomyopathy and hypercalcemia.
* In COPD, cough suppressing drugs are **contraindicated.**
* In asthmatic elderly patient with hypertension or angina, epinephrine is **contraindicated.**
* Morphine is avoided in patients with haemoptysis in Pulm. TB.
* Usual complication of pneumococcal pneumonia is Pleural effusion and that of Silicosis is TB.
* Metastatic lung lesions is caused by Staphylococcus

—Bronchiolitis in children	Ressp. Syncytial virus
—CROUP	Parainfluenza virus
—Thin walled cavity with pus	Coccidioidomycosis (pus in lung)
—Fungus ball in lung cavity	Aspergillosis
—Multiple cavities in lung	Blastomycosis
—Commonest Fungus infecting	

* The most common complication of whooping cough is asphyxia (expecially in infants-convulsion and brain damage)—Fairly common sequelae of pertusis is *Bronchiectasis.*
* **Obstructive Respiratory Disorders:** (Eg: *Chronic bronchitis and Emphysema)* have Lowered arterial pH during exacerbations;Increased PaCO2; Reduced PaO2 and SaO2; Reduced FVC, FEV1, MVV and PERR; Greater reduction in FEV1 than FVC; Increased RV and RV/TLC ratio; Increased non-elastic work of breathing; Uneven distribution of inspired gas.
* **Restrictive Respiratory Disorders :** (Eg: *Cryptogenic fibrosing alveolitis)* have Normal pH; Normal or low Pa CO2; Reduced Pa O2 and Sa O2; Decreased DLCO; Reduced FVC; Normal FEV/FVC ratio; Increased elastic work of breathing and decreased compliance; Slight impairment of gas distribution.
* **RESPIRATORY FAILURE**

Resp. Failure	:	Pa O2 < 8 k Pa
Type I	:	PaCO2 < 6.5 k Pa
Type II	:	PaCO2 > 6.5 k Pa

a. **Acute Type I** *(Severe hypoxaemia with a normal or low PaCO2) is caused by* Pulmonary oedema, Pneumonia, ARDS

b. **Chronic Type I** (*Chronic hypoxaemia without CO2 retention) is* caused by Fibrosing alveolitis, Interstitial lung diseases, Chronic pulmonary oedemma

c. **Acute Type II: (Asphyxia)** is caused by Upper airway obstruction (inhaled foreign body), Acute epiglottitis, Laryngeal oedema, Bilateral vocal cord palsy, Severe acute asthma, Chest acute asthma, Tension pneumothorax, Massive haemothorax, Flail chest, Brainstem and cervical cord lesions, Paralysis of resp. muscles, Narcotic poisoning

d. **Chronic Type II:** is caused by Chronic bronchitis, Progressive resp. disease.

* Drug of choice in emergency management of acute asthma — *Epinephrine and IV aminophylline*
* DOC in Status asthmaticus or acute attacks in epinephrine resistant patients — *IV hydrocortisone and methyl prednisolone (preperation of choice)*
* DOC in Klebsiella pneumonia is *Cephalothin (alternative-Gentamicin).*
* DOC in Legionella pneumonia is *Erythromycin*
* DOC in ***Pneumocystitis carinii*** pneumonia is *Sulfamethoxazole-trimethoprim* (alternative:pentamidine isothionate)
* DOC in Carcinoid lung is *Doxorubicin.*
* Persistent localised wheeze is an evidence of local bronchial obstruction.
* Pain in lung disease is due to involvement of parietal pleura. (Visceral pleura is insensitive to pain).
* Diaphargmatic irritation may cause pain referred to anterior shoulder (central irritation) or to upper abdomen (peripheral irritation).
* Haemoptysis with acute chest pain suggests pulmonary infarction.
* Collateral circulation between bronchial and pulmonary veins cause haemoptysis in mitral stenosis.
* Cyanosis represents increased concentration and reduced haemoglobin in the blood (**<5g/dL**).
* **Cyanosis** is less evident or does not occur in patients with hypoxia or histotoxic anaemia.
* Primary polycythaemia is usually associated with a normal arterial oxygen saturation.
* Aerosolized bronchodilator should be used to demonstrate potential reversibility of bronchospasm.
* Vital capacity with total lung capacity defines presence or absence or restrictive disease.
* Total lung capacity is usually greatly increased in obstructive disease.
* Best single measurement of ability to cough is forced expiratory flow **(200-1200 L/min).**
* Reduced forced expiratory flow in 1 second (FEVI) suggests obstruction.

* $PaCO_2$ is the most reliable assessment of adequacy of ventilation.
* **Heimlich procedure** is especially applicable with obstruction due to an inhaled bolus of food.
* Obstruction to air flow during both inspiratory and expiratory phases occurs in fixed tracheal obstruction.
* Tuberculin and various fungus antigen skin tests are usually negative even when these infections are present in sarcoidosis.
* The patient in sarcoidosis is relatively asymptomatic even in the presence of obvious clinical disease.
* Renal failure due to glomerulitis and pulmonary failure is the usual cause of death in Wegner's granulomatosis.
* Eosinophilia usually does not occur in extrensic allergic alveolitis (Hypersensitivity pneumonitis).
* *Herpes simplex* facial lesions are often present in pneumococcal pneumonia.
* **Pseudocavitation** is seen in pneumococcal pneumonia.
* Bullae of varying sizes may be seen in
  (i) Upper lung fields — chronic bronchitis
  (ii) Lower lung fields — Emphysema
* **Pink puffers** (emphysema) denotes predominant panacinar emphysema (deficiency of alpha 1 antitrypsin).
* **Blue bloaters** (chronic bronchitis)—centrilobular emphysema (cigerette smoking irritant inhalations).
* The only symptom may be relatively sudden onset of dyspnea with or without pleuritic chest pain is associated with pulmonary embolism.
* **Pulmonary angiography** is necessary for the definitive diagnosis of clinically significant pulmonary emboli.
* The presence of calcification in solitary pulmonary nodule is strong evidence against pulm. malignancy.
* Reduction in cardiac output is one of the most significant side effects of PEEP.
* The optimal level of PEEP is the pessure just below that at which cardiac output becomes reduced.
* The **adult respiratory distress syndrome** (ARDS) has been defined clinically by the **triad** of (i) refractory hypoxemia, (ii) decreased lung compliance, and (iii) diffuse alveolar infiltrates once a stable chronic pulmonary process and hydrostatic pulmonary edema have been excluded. ARDS usually presents clinically as tachypnea and laboured breathing, reflecting a reduced lung compliance. Arterial blood gases generally reveal preserved ventilation with profound hypoxemmia resistant to supplement oxygen.

- Anaerobic lung infection results from aspiration of polymicrobial oropharyngeal flora.
- Treatmment of choice for anaerobic pleuropulmonary infection is penicillin G or clindamycin; cefoxitin is an acceptable alternative consideration, as is metronidazole.
- Empyema requires thoracostomy tube drainage; lung abscess rarely requires surgical resection.
- **Acute respiratory failure** is defined as:
  1. $PaO2 \leq 50$ mmHg *or*
  2. $PaCO2 \geq 50$ mmHg and arterial $pH \leq 7.35$
- In Ac. Resp. failure, **mechanical ventilation** is indicated for:
  1. $PaO2 \leq 40$ with respiratory acidosis and altered mental status
  2. Failure of conservative therapy to correct hypxoemia without unacceptable worsening of respiratory acidosis.
  3. Incipient respiratory muscle fatigue:
     a. Increasing respiratory rate
     b. Respiratory alternans
     c. Abdominal paradox
  4. Inability of patient to expectorate copious airway secretions
- The parietal pleura lines the thoracic cage, mediastinum, and superior surface of the diaphragm; is only loosely adherent; and has a systemic blood supply and **innervation.**
- Exudative effusions are defined by the following:
  1. Pleural fluid protein/serum protein >5, *or*
  2. Pleural fluid LDH/serum $\geq .6$, *or*
  3. Pleural fluid LDH above two to three times upper limit of normal serum LDH.
- Grossly bloody pleural effusions generaly result from trauma, malignancy, or pulmonary embolism.
- A predominance of polymorphonuclear leukocytes in an exudative effusion suggests acute infection or other inflammatory processes.
- Eosinophils and basophils are nondiagnostic; plasma cells in pleural fluid are associated with plasma cell dyscrasias.
- **Low pleural fluid glucose** concentration usually occurs in the clinical settings of infection, rheumatoid arthritis, tuberculosis, or malignancy.
- Fluid complement levels and an LE preparation may substantiate the diagnosis of connective tissue disease; rheumatoid factor is nondiagnostic.
- Increased **pleural fluid amylase** levels suggest pancreatitis, esophageal rupture or malignancy.

* The diagnosis of pleural malignancy or tuberculosis may require pleural biopsy.
* **Pneumothorax** most commonly arises spontaneously from rupture of a visceral pleural bleb in an otherwise healthy young person.
* Pneumothorax may also occur in association with trauma, or complicate diagnostic procedures.
* All pneumothoraces ≥ 15-30% of the hemithorax volume or of any extent during positive pressure ventilation require closed chest tube thoracostomy.
* **Fibrothorax** generally occurs as a complication of previous empyema or hemothorax and may necessitate decorti- cation.
* **Metastatic involvement of the pleura** occurs most commonly with carcinomas of the breast, lung, or ovary, and with lymphomas.
* Benign mesotheliomas usually present as isolated mass lesions of the visceral pleura.
* **Graham steel murmur** is heard in Pulmonary incompetence due to Pulm. hypertension.
* After surgery for VSD the frequent conduction defect seen in RBBB.
* A fancy name given for chronic constrictive pericarditis is **Pick's disease.**
* **Adson's test** is for *Thoracic outlet syndrome.*
* **Escherich's test** is a modification of tuberculin reaction.
* **Flack test** is for Respiratory efficiency
* **Hamburger's test** is type of tuberculin test.
* **Lignieres' test** is a cutaneous reaction with tuberculin for TB.
* Pleural pain is usually unilateral, aggravated by changes in intrathoracic pressure (cough, sneeze, deep breathing).
* In oesophageal irritation or spasm pain is deep and central, altered by swallowing.
* Cyanosis is less evident or does not occur in Pts. with **hypoxia** due to anemia or histotoxic hypoxia (presence or absence of hypoxemia should be confirmed by measuring O2 tension of arterial blood).
* Calcifications of diaphragmatic pleura are especially characteristic of asbestosis.
* Trachea is **central** in **pneumonic consolidition.**
* Valvular pneumothorax is a medical emergency.
* **Slient asthma** is a more serious than noisy asthma.
* Primary complex can occur in adults.
* Open pneumothorax is associated with **amphoric breathing.**
* Tetany can produce laryngeal stridor is infants.

* **Adson's test** is for Thoracic outlet syndrome
* **Escherich's test** is a type of tuberculin test.
* **Lignieres' test** is a cutaneous reaction with tuberculin for TB.
* Peripheral neuropathy can occur in carcinoma lung.
* Miliary tuberculosis is confirmed by demonstrating AFB in sputum.
* Asbestosis produces a restrictive lung defect.
* Pleural mesothelioma will produce pneumothorax.
* Tuberculin test may be negative in miliary tuberculosis.
* Trachea is central in pneumonic consolidation.
* Extrinsic asthma is common in childhood.
* Disodium chromoglycate is a bronchodilator.
* Aspirin sensitivity is a feature of intrinsic asthma.
* Silicosis predisposes to the development of tuberculosis.
* In intrinsic bronchial asthma, there is strong family history.
* FEV is normal in status asthmaticus.
* **Pulsus paradoxus** can occur in tension pneumothorax.
* Disodium chromoglycate cures an attack of bronchial asthma.
* Corticosteroids flare up dormant tuberculosis.
* Hypercapnia is a feature of restrictive lung disease.
* All that wheezes is **not** a bronchial asthma.
* Silent asthma is a more serious than noisy asthma.
* Trachea gets pulled to same side in fibrosis.
* Bronchogenic carcinoma may present as unresolved pneumonia.
* Diphragm moves freely in pleural effusion.
* Hydrothorax can occur in C.C.F.
* Anaerobic bacteria frequently produce pneumonia.
* Oxygen administration improves central cyanosis in pulmonary condition.
* Primary complex can occur in adults.
* Trachea gets pulled to same side in consolidation.
* Bronchogenic carcinoma can produce **Cushing's syndrome.**
* Sputum for AFB is positive in disseminated primary complex.
* Primary atypical pneumonia is produced by H. influenza organisms.
* With modern chemotherapy, the duration of treatment of tuberculosis is reduced to nearly **9 months.**
* Extrimities are warm in peripheral cyanosis.
* Open pneumothorax is associated with amphoric breathing.

* Tension pneumothorax is treated by emergency insertion of needle.
* Pulmonary osteoarthropathy is usually due to carcinoma lung.
* IgE type of immunoglobulin is involved in causing an attack of bronchial asthma.
* In pneumococcal pneumonia, the drug of choice is crystalline penicillin.
* Recent tuberculin converter should get INH as chemoprophylaxis agent.
* **Commonest** cause of haemorrhagic pleural effusion inelderly male is carcinoma lung.
* The **Drug of choice** in the treatment of tropical eosinophilia is diethylcarbamazine.
* Absent breath sounds with pull of mediastinum to the same side suggest collapse.
* Anaerobic bacterial pneumonias are treated with metronidazole.
* Carcinoid syndrome, a malignant disease may manifest as bronchial asthma.
* Hemoptysis may occur in metastatic carcinoma of lung.
* Behcet's syndrome has an association with **HLA-B5.**
* Hilar adenopathy is not a feature of lipid pneumonia.
* Silicosis is seen in mining, stone cutting, sandblasting, and foundry work. Asbestosis is associated with mining. milling, shipyard work, and insulation work.
* **Silicotic nodules** become calcified in the upper lung lobes.
* Carbon dioxide retention is seen in right-to-left shunt only with exercise and is uncommon in impaired diffusion syndromes.
* Granulomatous inflammatory changes of sarcoidosis may occur in almost any organ.
* The Kveim test requires **six weeks** incubation.
* Acute granulomatous uveitis may be the initial manifestation of sarcoidosis.
* In bronchiectasis the posterior basal segments of the lower lobes are likely to be the **most commonly** involved area. True bronchiectasis is not reversible.
* **Drug of choice** for exercise induced asthma is Ipratropium.
* **Most characteristic** lesion seen in asbestosis is pleural plaques.
* In massive pulmonary embolism, the embolus may obstruct pulmonary veins.
* A patient suffering from lung abscess develops anasarca. The probabale reason is **amyloidosis.**

* Recurrent aspiration pneumonia is caused by progressive systemic sclerosis.
* Respiratory symptoms are associated with Strongyloidiasis.
* Non respiratory function of lung is **Serotonin metabolism.**
* Longterm complication of bronchopulmonary dysplasia is small airway disease.
* In an asymptomatic smoker one would find ↑ closing volume.
* Wedge pressure in ARDS is usually normal.
* Wide alveolar arterial O2 gradient is seen in bronchiectasis, ARDS and Interstitial fibrosis.
* Respiration may occur in foetus delivered at 18th week.
* For persistent hypoxia (PaO2<50 mm Hg) or for severe hypercapnia (PaCO2> 60 mm Hg), intubation and mechanical ventilation are indicated
* In uncomplicated pneumothorax, the extrapulmonary air will usually resolve in 24-48 hours.
* The use of 100% oxygen, while effective in speeding the resolution of pneumothorax, is not recommended in premature infants because of the danger of retinopathy of prematuity and possible pulmonary toxicity.
* The **most frequent** medical problem in childhood is common cold.
* The **most common** chronic lung disease of children is Asthma.
* The **most common** trigger for asthma attack in young children is respirataory viral infection.
* The **commonest** cause of fever in children is due to upper respiratory tract infection.
* The **most common** lethal inherited disease of Caucasians is cystic fibrosis.
* The **most common** cause of stridor in infancy is Laryngomalacia (infantile larynx)
* The **most common** congenital laryngeal abnormality is Laryngomalacia.
* Commonest cause of Haematemesis — Acute duodenal ulcer
* Commonest cause of bronchiolitis — Respiratory syncytial virus
* Commonest cause of epiglottitis — H. influenzae
* Commonest cause of croup — Parainfluenza virus type I
* Commonest cause of Empyema — Staphylococci
* Commonest cause of Pleural/Pericardialeffusion — TB
* Commonest cause of Constrictive Pericarditis — TB
* Cystic firbrosis is probably the **most common** childhood cause of nasal polyposis.
* The condition **most commonly** confused with acute bronchiolitis is bronchial asthma.

* **Most common cause** of pneumonia in childhood is due to viral infection
* The **most common** bacterial pathogen causing childhood bacterial penumonia is Streptococcus penumoniae (over 90%). Viral pneumonia is **most commonly** caused by Respiratory syncytial viral.
* The **most common** forms of pulmonary malgnancy in childhood is due to Metastatic lesions **(such** as Wilm's tumour, osteogenic sarcoma & Hepatoblastoma).
* The **most common** cause of pneumomediastinum in older children & teenagers in Acute asthma.
* Staphylococcus aureus is the **most commonly** isolated pathogen from bacterial tracheitis.
* Cystic fibrosis is the **most common** underlying disease in children with generalized bronchial involment of bronchiectasis.
* An arterial blood gas analysis is probably the single **most useful** test of pulmonary function.
* Most common cause of bacterial meningitis...

  - in neonates ... group B streptococci & E coli
* The principal pulmonary surfactant is a specialised phospholipid (dipalmitoyl lecithin or phosphatidyl choline) synthesized by Type II alveolar cells (Pneumocytes)
* Reversible bronchiectasis or pseudobronchiectasis occurs commonly after perfussis, lobar & interstitial penumonias.
* Bicarbonate should not be administered in a patient with impending respiratory failure.
* **Silofiller's disease** is an acute interstitial pneumonia occurs following the inhalation of nitrogen dioxide.
* **Ehlers-Danlos disease & Marfan syndrome** are unusually prone to develop pneumothorax.
* **Head-bobing** is a sign of dyspnea is an exhausted or sleeping infant.
* Virtually all men with cystic fibrosis are sterile whereas women are fertile
* Most recurrent or persistent wheezing in children is the result of reactive airway disease
* When plurisy & pneumonia continue for more than 2 wk, tuberculosis should be considered.
* Hydrothorax is usually bilateral in nutritional edema & renal disease and in myocardinal disease it is limited to the right side.
* Subcutaneous emphysema, if present, is virtually diagnostic of pneumomediastinum.
* Croup syndrome is associated with Parainfluenza virus.

* Pharyngitis with conjunctivits is most often by Adenovirus.
* The earliest symptom of cystic fibrosis may be cough.
* The retropharynx in retropharyngeal abscess should not be palpated because of the risk of rupture, aspiration or mediastinitis, and death.
* Theophylline toxicity includes severe headache, tachycardia, tremors, gastritis with frequent vomiting, and seizures.
* Apnea is common in preterm infants.
* **Silverman's scoring** is done to assess respiratory distress.
* High aiway resistance in a child increases risk of devleoping obstructive lung disease.
* Intercostal retractions suggest cystic fibrosis.
* Pulmonary function tests are difficult in children with tracheostomies.
* A small increase in respiratory rate and a marked increased in respiratory effort may occur, particularly in inspiration producing a harsh low pitched inspiratory sound called Stridor.
* The etiological agent associated with bronchiolitis obliterans and unilateral hyperlucent lung syndrome (Suyer James syndrome) is Adenovirus.
* A definite diagnosis of tracheal foreign body can be made only by Bronchoscopy.
* Increase of stridor when a child is supine suggests laryngomalacia/ tracheomalacia
* An uncommon but characteristic syndrome appearing in the first year of life with recurrent lung infilterates is pulmonary haemosiderosis related to cow's milk hypersensitivity.
* Encapsulated pleural effusion in X-ray is seen as convex border.
* Too high oxygen concentration can cause pulmonary oedema.
* Pure left sided heart failure is seen with PDA
* The commonest cause of corpulmonale in children in cystic fibrosis
* Delayed respiratory distress syndrome is seen in **Wilson Mikity syndrome**
* In pneumonia, of pulse pressure in mm Hg does not fall below the pulse rate, the prognosis is good it is **Gibson's rule**
* A redline observed on the gingivae in pulmonary tuberculosis is **Thompson's line**
* In esophageal atresia, pneumonia is most common in right upper lobe
* If respiratory distress does not appear within **12-18 hours,** then hyaline membrance disease is unlikely
* **Commonest** clinical presentation of certain important tumors:
* Bronchogenic tumors—shortness of breath/cough.

* **"Egg shell calcification"** in lung is seen characteristically in silicosis.
* **"Meniscus sign"** in lung is most commonly seen in aspergillus fungus ball.
* **Anterior Mediastinal Masses** ("Four Ts")
  Thyroid, Thymoma, Teratoma, T-cell Lymphoma (Hodgkin's)
* **Middle Mediaslium** : Aneurysm, LN, Oesophageal duplication cysts, Branchogenic cyst, Pericardial cyst
* **Posterior Mediastinal masses** Neurogenic masses (schwannomas, Pheochromocytoma, chemodectoma, meningocele)
* **Lung Tumours**
  - Most common among smokers)
    Squamous cell
  - Most common (among non-smokers
    Adenocarcinoma
    and females)
  - Least Common — Large cell type
  - Worst prognosis — Small cell type
  - Most common Scar Carcinoma
    Adeno carcinoma
  - Most frequent to Cavitate

Pleural effusion:

* **Bacelli's Sign**
  — Good conducttion of the whisper in non purulent pleural effusions
* **D' Amato's Sign**
  — Position of dullness is altered from vertebral area in sitting position to heart region when patient assumes a lateral position on the opposite side of effusion.
* **Ellis's Sign**
  — S-shaped line of dullness over chest, highest in axilla and lower in anterior and posterior part
* **Grocco's Sign**
  — Triangular area of dullness on the back of opposite side of effusion
* **Karplus' Sign**
  — On auscultation over effusion vowel 'U' spoken by patient is heard as 'A' (due to modification in vocal resonance)

* **Kellock's Sign**
  — Increase of vibration of ribs on sharp percussion with Rt. hand, and Lt. hand being placed firmly on thorax
* **Koranyi's Sign**
  — Increase in resonance over dorsal segment on percussion of spinal process of thoracic vertabrae.
* **Sicar's Sign**
  — Metallic resonance is heard on percussion with two coins on front of the chest and auscultation at the back.
* **William's Sign**
  — Dullness over second intercostal space

Pneumothorax with Pleural effusion:

* **Hoover's Sign**
  — Movement of costal margins toward midline in inspiration - Bilaterally in pulmonary emphysema and unilaterally in pleural effusion and pneumothorax
* **Williamson's Sign**
  — Markedly diminished BP in leg as compared with thaat in the arm on the same side.

Pneumonia with Pleural Effusion:

* **Skoda's Sign**
  — Tympanitic note heard on percussion of chest above the level of pleural effusion

Pleurisy:

* **Andral's Sign** (early stages of pleurisy)
  — patient prefers to lie on same side
* **Ramond's Sign** (pleurisy with pleural effusion)
  — rigidity of the erector spinae muscles
* **Schepelimann's Sign** (Dry pleurisy)
  — increased pain when patient bends his body towards normal side
* **Spinal Sign**
  — Tonic contraction of spinal muscles on diseased side

Cavity of lung:

* **Seitz's Sign**
  — On inspiration bronchial sound is heard which begins harshly and then becomes faint
* **Wintrich's Sign**
  — Change in the pitch of percussion note when mouth is opened and closed

Bronchial gland enlargement:

* **Schick's Sign (in infants)**
  — Stridor heard on inspiration
* **Smith Sign**
  — murmur heard over manubrium on ausculatation when patients, head is thrown back (due to pressure of glands on innominate veins)

Pulmonary tuberculosis:

* **Abraham's Sign** (early apical TB)
  — Percussion note is dull and flat over acromian process
* **Riviere's Sign**
  — A change in percussion not e denoting a band of increased density across the back at the plane of spinous process if 5th, 6th and 7th dorsal vertebrae

Infantile pneumonia:

* **Weill's Sign**
  — Absence of expansion in sub-clavicular region on the affected side.

Hydropneumothorax:

* **Biermer's Sign**
  — Shifting metallic resonance with change of position

Fibrous mediastinitis:

* **Perez's Sign**
  — rales audible over upper part of chest when arms are alternately raised and lowered (also seen in aneurysm of aortic arch)

Hydatid cyst of lung:

* **Bird's Sign**
  — Presence of a zone of dullness on percussion with absence of resp. sounds at the site of hydatid cyst

Paralysis of diaphragm:

* **Duchenne's Sign**
  — Sinking of epigastrium on inspiration

Tracheal stenosis:

* **Aufrech's Sign**
  — Feelble breath sounds heard just above the jugular fossa
* **Ayerza's Syndrome**
  Etiology: Sec. to primary disease to pulm. artery (due to *syphilis* and *pulm. arteriolar sclerosis*)

  Dyspnea, cyanosis, polycythemia, slowly developing asthma and bronchitis

* **Brock's (middle lobe) Syndrome**

  Obstruction of middle lobe bronchus by mucous plugs or tubercular lymphnodes, cause collapse of middle lobe and is seen in childhood. Recurrent pneumonia, productive cough and haemoptysis

* **Caplan's Syndrome**

  Rheumatoid arthritis and coal workers pneumoconiosis

  — Round, well demarcated lesions in lungs (intrapulmonary nodules)

* **Hamman-rich Syndrome**

  Ac. or chr. interstitial fibrosis of lung

  — Arterial hypoxemia, cyanosis, right sided heart failure and cor pulmonale

* **Kartagener's Syndromme**

  AD or AR — chronic sinusitis, bronchiectasis and situs inverssus

  Others: recurrent pneumonia, undeveloped frontal sinus, myopia, glaucoma, retinal pigmentary degeneration

* **Leredde's syndrome**

  Congenital syphilis — severe dyspnoea on exertion with advanced emphysema, recurrent attacks of ac. febrile bronchitis (from early childhood)

* **Loeffler's Syndrome**

  Reagin mediated hypersensitivity seen with *Ascariaasis, Ancylostomiasis, strongloides cutaneous larva migrans, drugs, periarteritis nodosa* and *inhaled allergens.*

  — transient pulmonary infiltration with eosinophilia associated with fever, cough, breathlessness, anorexia and weight loss

* **Meigs' Syndrome**

  Unknown — fibromyoma of ovary (rarely Brenner's tumour) with ascites and hydrothorax (right sided pleural effusion)

* **Pancoast's-Milkity Syndrome** (Hare syndrome)

  Involvement of brachial plexus due to apical carcinoma of lung

  — pain in arm, shoulder and interscapular region, wasting of small muscles of hand on corresponding side with sensory disturbances in arm and hand, and ipsilateral Horner's Syndrome.

* **Wilson-Mikity Syndrome**

(Pulmonary dysmaturity syndrome)

Unknown (seen in *premaature infants <32 wks. of gestation)* — Lungs contain wide spread focal emphysematous blebs and parenchymma thickened alveolar walls. Fever, wheezing and rales with right sided heart failure

RESPIRATORY SYSTEM

COMMON RESPIRATORY DISEASES BY DIAGNOSTIC CATEGORIES

Obstructive

Asthma

Chronic obstructive lung disease (chronic bronchitis, emphysema)

Bronchiectasis

Cystic fibrosis

Bronchiolitis

Restrictive—parenchymal

Sarcoidosis

Idiopathic pulmonary fibrosis

Pneumoconiosis

Drug or radiation-induced interstitial lung disease

Restrictive—extraparenchymal

Neuromuscular

- Diaphragmatic weakness/paralysis
- Myasthenia gravis*
- Guillain-Barre syndrome*
- Muscular dystrohies*
- Cervical spine injury*

Chest wall

- Kyphoscoliosis
- Obesity
- Ankylosing spondylitis*

* Can have inspiratory and expiratory limitation

INDICATIONS FOR BRONCHOSCOPY

Indication	*Comments*
Diagnostic	
Hemoptysis	Best performed when bleeding has almost stopped
Chronic unexplained cough	May be early manifestation of endobronchial tumor
Undiagnosed mass	Transbronchial biopsy may be performed
Delayed resolution of pneumonia	Excludes bronchial obstruction as cause
Localized atelectasis	Identify cause of bronchial obstruction of present
Evaluate operability in lung cancer can be assessed	Extent of proximal spread and node involvement
Positive sputum cytology with negative x-ray	Fiberoptic scope will permit localization of nearly all occult lung cancer
Lung abscess	Exclude bronchial obstruction, obtain material for culture.
Tracheal extubation	Evaluate trauma to airway resulting from intubation
Therapeutic	
Control of hemorrhage	Endobronchial lesion may occasionally be cauterized.
Removal of foreign body	Rigid bronchoscope preferred
Lobar atelectasis in patient on respirator	Aspiration of secretions through bronchoscope permits reexpansion
Lung abscess which drains poorly	Repeated endoscopy may promote drainage

SOME CAUSES OF HYPERCAPNIA (RAISED PaCO)

Central	*Chest wall*
Brain-stem lesions	Kyphoscoliosis
Central sleep apnoea	Ankylosing spondylitis
	Trauma
Neuromuscular	
Peripheral neuropathy	Pulmonary
Myasthenia gravis	Chronic bronchitis
Myopathies	(and emphysema)

CAUSES OF HYPOXAEMIA

* Venous admixture effect (poorly ventilated lung)	
* Alveolar underventilation (raised $PaCO_2$)	Corrected by oxygen

* Impairment of diffusion (less important at rest)
* Right-to-left shunts (circulatory channels bypassing lungs)
* Reduced oxygen content ($PaCO_2$ may be normal) (anaemia, inactivated haemoglobin)

TYPES OF COUGH (WITH SOME EXAMPLES)

Freely productive	Bronchiectasis
Paroxysmal	Chronic bronchitis, asthma
Painful	Pneumonia with pleurisy
'Bovine' (lacking explosive element)	Recurrent laryngeal paralysis
Accompanied by stridor	Whooping cough; partial laryngeal or tracheal obstruction

TYPES OF SPUTUM

White	Mucoid
Gray	Mucoid (dust inhalation)
Black	Mucoid + coal dust (melanoptysis)
Yellow or green	Purulent
Rusty	Altered blood (pneumococcal pneumonia)
Pink frothy	Pulmonary oedema
Blood-stained	Haemoptysis

CAUSES OF HAEMOPTYSIS

* Pulmonary tuberculosis
* Bronchial tumours (carcinoma, adenoma)
* Pulmonary infarction
* Bronchiectasis
* Mitral stenosis

CAUSES OF FINGER CLUBBING

Respiratory	*Non-respiratory*
Bronchial carcinoma	Cyanotic congenital heart disease
Chronic intrathoracic suppuration (e.g. bronchiectasis,	Infective endocarditis
lung abscess; empyema)	Crohn's disease
Fibrosing alveolitis	Malabsorption syndrome
Asbestosis	Hepatic cirrhosis
	Familial trait

RESPIRATORY FAILURE

Definition

$PaO_2 < 8.0$ kPa (60 mmHg) and/or
$PaCO_2 > 6.5$ kPA (50 mm Hg)

Type 1

PaO_2 low $PaCO_2$ normal or low

Type II

$PaCO_2$ raised PaO_2 low-'ventilatory failure'

SYMPTOMS OF POST-PRIMARY TUBERCULOSIS

Cough

May be early symptom but often not troublesome until a late stage

Sputum

Only when disease has reached an advanced stage. Mucoid at first; later purulent

Haemoptysis

Common when disease advanced. May be massive from a large vessel in a cavity wall; sometimes fatal

Breathlessness

Late symptom unless caused bypenumothorax when onset is acute

Pleural pain

Can be due to tuberculous pleurisy, but occasionally

Pneumothorax

SYMPTOMS AND SIGNS WHICH SHOULD ALWAYS RAISE THE SUSPICION OF TB

* Persistent cough
* Haemoptysis
* Pleural pain not associated with an acute illness
* Spontaneous pneumothorax
* Lethargy
* Weight loss

DIAGNOSTIC FEATURES OF ALLERGIC BRONCHOPULMONARY ASPERGILLOSIS (ABPA)

MAIN DIAGNOSTIC CRITERIA

1. Bronchial asthma
2. Pulmonary infiltrates
3. Peripheral eosinophilia (> 1000 per cubic microliter)
4. Immediate wheal and flare response to *Aspergillus fumigatus*
5. Serum precipitins to A. *funigatus*
6. Elevated serum IgE
7. Central bronchiectasis

OTHER DIAGNOSTIC FEATURES

1. History of brownish plugs in sputum
2. Culture of A. fumigatus from sputum
3. Elevated IgE (and IgG) class antibodies specific for A. fumigatus

CAUSES OF BRONCHIECTASIS

Congenital

Ciliary dysfunction syndromes, cystic fibrosis, primary hypogammaglobulinaemia

Acquired

Pheumonia (whooping cough and measles), primary tuberculosis, foreign body

Adults

Suppurative pneumonia, pulmonary tuberculosis, pulmonary eosinphilia, bronchial tumours

SYMPTOMS OF BRONCHIECTASIS

Due to accumulation of pus in dilated bronchi

Chronic productive cough usually worse in mornings and often brought on by changes of posture. Sputum often copious and persistently purulent in advanced disease.

Due to inflammatory changes in lung and pleura surrounding dilated bronchi

Fever, malaise and increased cough and sputum volume when spread of infection causes penumonia, which is frequently associted withpleurisy. Recurrent pleurisy in the same site often occurs in bronchiectasis

Haemoptysis

Can be slight or massive and is often recurrent. Usually associated with purulent sputum or an increase in sputum purulence. Can, however, be the only symptom in so-called '*dry bronchiectasis*'

General health

When disease is extensive and sputum perisistently purulent a decline in gneral health occurs with weight loss, anorexia, lassitude, sleep sweating and failure to thrive in children. In these patients, finger clubbing is common.

CHRONIC OBSTRUCTIVE LUNG DISEASE: SALIENT FEATURES OF THE TWO TYPES

	Predominant emphysema	*Predominant bronchitis*
Age at time of diagnosis (Years)	60 ±	50
Dyspnea	Severe	Mild
Cough	After dyspnea starts	Before dyspnea starts
Sputum	Scanty, mucoid	Copious, purulent
Bronchial infections	Less frequent	More frequent
Respiratory insufficiency episodes	Often terminal	Repeated
Chest film	"Hyperinflation" * bullous changes, small heart	Increased bronchovascular markings at bases, large heart
Chronic PaCO2, mmHg	35-40	50-60
Chronic PaO2, mm Hg	65-75	45-60
Pulmonary hypertension :		
Rest	None to mild	Moderate to severe
Exercise	Moderate	Worse
Cor pulmonale	Rare, except terminally	
Elastic recoil	Severely decreased	Normal
Resistance	Normal to slight increase	High
Diffusing capacity	Decreased	Normal to slight decrease

PRINCIPAL CLINICAL MANIFESTATIONS OF CYSTIC FIBROSIS

I *Respiratory/cardiovascular*

A. Bronchitis, bronchopneumonia, bronchiectasis, lung abscess, aspergillosis (allergic)

B. Atelectasis

C. Sinusitis, nasal polyposis

D. Pulmonary hypertension

E. Cor pulmonale and congestive heart failure

F. Hemoptysis

G. Penumothorax

H. Respiratory failure

II. *Gastrointestinal*

A. Intestinal

1. Meconium ileus
2. Volvulus
3. Ileal atresia
4. Rectal prolapse
5. Intussuception
6. Fecal impaction
7. Pneumatosis intestinalis

B. Pancreatic

1. Nutritional deficit and growth failure due to pancreatic insufficiency
2. Steatorrhea
3. Diabetes mellitus
4. Recurrent pancreatitis

C. Hepatobiliary

1. Atrophic gallbladder, cholelithiasis
2. Loss of bile salts
3. Focal biliary cirrhosis
4. Portal hypertension
   a. Esophageal varices
   b. Hypersplenism
   c. Hemorrhoids

III. ***Reproductive system***

A. Males : sterility ; absent or defective vas deferens, epididymis, and seminal vesicles in about 99 percent of males

B. Females : decreased fertility; increased viscosity of vaginal secretions

IV. ***Skeletal***

A. Retardation of bone age

B. Demineralization

C. Hypertrophic osteoarthropathy

V. ***Other***

A. Salt depletion

B. Heat stroke

C. Salivary gland hypertrophy

D. Retinal hemorrhage

E. Hypertrophy of apocrine glands

CAUSES OF INTERSTITIAL LUNG DISEASE

* Chronic pulmonary oedema e.g. secondary to mitral valve disease
* Extrinsic allergic alveolitis
* Cryptogenic fibrosing alveolitis and fibrosing alveolitis associated with connective tissue disorders
* Pulmonary damage following radiotherapy to the lungs
* Drugs, e.g. bleomycin, busulphan, methotrexate, amiodarone, gold, nitrofurantoin, paraquat
* Sarcoidosis
* Asbestosis
* Idiopathic pulmonary haemosiderosis

OCCUPATIONS ASSOCIATED WITH SILICOSIS

* Mining-coal, tin, gold, other minerals
* Quarrying
* Dressing of sandstone and granite
* The pottery and cramics industry
* Manufacture of silica blocks and abrasive soaps
* Iron and steel industries
* Sand-blasting
* Boiler scaling

PLEURO-PULMONARY DISORDERS CAUSED BY INHALATION OF ASBESTOS

* Benign pleural plaques
* Benign pleural effusion
* Progressive pulmonary fibrosis (asbestosis)
* Malignant disease of the pleura (mesothelioma)

PULMONARY CHANGES IN SARCOIDOSIS

Stage I

X-ray shows bilateral hilar enlargement, usually symmetrical; paratracheal nodes often enlarged

Spontaneous resolution usually within one year in majority of cases. Often asymptomatic, but may be associated with erythema nodosum and arthralgia

Stage II

X-ray shows a combination of hilar glandular enlargement and pulmonary opacities which are often diffuse, but not always.

Patients usually asymptomatic. Spontaneous improvement occurs in majority.

Stage III

X-ray shows diffuse pulmonary shadows without evidence of hilar adenopathy. Evidence of pulmonary fibrosis may be present or develop.

Disease less likely to resolve spontaneously. Pulmonary fibrosis can cause breathlessness, pulmonary hypertension and cor pulmonale.

EXTRA-PULMONARY MANIFESTATIONS OF SARCOIDOSIS

Eyes

Phlyclenular conjunctivitis; uveitis; iridocycilits; lacrimal gland involvement

Skin

Erythema nodosum, cutaneous 'sarcoids' (skinpapules), infiltration of scars; lupus pernio-red/blue infiltration of nose, cheeks and ear lobes.

Salivary glands

Parotid gland enlargement. Can cause facial palsy. May be associated with eye involvement and fever ('uveoparotid fever').

Heart
Myocarditis; conduction defects
Kidneys
Nephrocalcinosis
Liver and spleen
Enlargement caused by granulomatous infiltration. Usually asymptomatic. Hypersplenism rarely
Nervous system
Cerebral, meningeal, cranial and peripheral nerve involvement
Bones and joints
Arthralgia; arthritis; phalangeal cysts

DRUG INTERACTIONS OF THEOPHYLLINE

* **↓ Theophyllinel Plasma levels levels (By ↑ metabolism)**
  - Smoking
  - Phenytoin
  - Rifampicin
  - Phenobarb
  - Charcoal broiled meal milk
* **↑ Theophylline Plasma (By ↓ metabolism)**
  - Erythromycin
  - Ciprofloxacin
  - Cimetidine
  - OCP
  - Allopurinol
  - * (decrease dose to 2/3)
* **Theophylline ↑ effects of**
  - Furosemide
  - Sympathomimetics
  - Digitalis
  - Oral anticoagulants
* **↓ es effects of**
  - Phenytoin
  - Lithium

* **Aminophylline injection should not be mixed in same infusion bottle/syringe with —**
  ascorbic acid, chlorpromazine, promethazine, morphine, pethidine, pethidine, phenytoin, phenobarb, insulin, penicillin G, tetracyclines, erythromycin

* RESPIRATORY MANIFESTATIONS

A. Airway obstruction
(bronchopasm, asthma)
Beta blockers
Cephalosporines

Cholinergic drugs
Nonsteroidal antiinflammatory drugs e.g. aspirin, indomethacin
Penicillins
Pentazocine
Streptomycin
Tartrazine (drugs with yellow dye)

B. Cough

Angiotensin-converting enzyme inhibitors

C. Nasal congestion

Decongestant abuse
Guanethidine
Isoproterenol
Oral contraceptives

D. Pulmonary edema

Contrast media
Heroin
Hydrochlorthiazide
Methadone
Propoxyphene

E. Pulmonary infiltrates

Amiodarone
Azothioprine
Bleomycin
Busulfan
Carmustine (BCNU)
Chlorambucil
Cyclophosphamide
Melphalan
Methotrexate
Methysergide
Mitomycin C
Nitrofurantoin
Procarbaxzine
Sulfonamides

F. Respiratory depression

Aminoglycosides
Hypnotics
Opiates
Polymyxins
Sedatives
Trimethaphan

RESPIRATORY VARIABLE IN THE NEONATE

Tital Volume (Vt)	7 ml/kg
Dead space (Vd)	Vr X 0.3 ml
Respiratory rate	Age 1-3 (24..age/2)breath/min

* COMPARISON OF RESPIRATORY VARIABLES IN NEWBORNS, INFANTS, CHILDREN AND ADULTS

Age	Weight (Kg.)	Respirataory Rate (breaths/min	Tidal Volume (ml)	Minute Ventilation (ml/min)	FRC (ml)	VC (ml)	Vd (ml)
Newborn	3	35	15	525	70	90	7
6 months	6	30	30	900	150	200	14
12 months	10	24	70	1,680	260	470	21
5 years	18	20	135	2,700	660	1,100	49
23 years	70	12	500	6,000	3,000	4,600	150

Abbreviations: FRC, functional residual capacity, VC, vital capacity: Vd, respiratory dead space

LOEFFLER SYNDROME:

* Allergic manifestation
* Widespread transitory pulmonary infiltrations
* Blood eosinophilia (70%)
* Paroxysmal attacks of coughing, dyspnea, pleurisy & little or no fever
* Hepatomegaly in infants & young children
* Hyperglobulinemia
* Localized pneumonic consolidation with associated eosinophilia
* Most common pathogen is the Toxocara canis

CHEST

A. Coin Shaped (Solitary Cricrumscribed Nodules)

* Granulomas-Tuberculosis, Histoplasmosis, Coccidiodomycosis
* Cyst-bronchial, Hydatid
* Bronchial Adenoma

* Hamartomas
* Bronchogenic carcinoma
* Metastatic Nodule
* Chest wall Lesions-Mesothelioma or Fibroma of Pleura
* Others-Subpleural lymph nodes, Pneumonia, A V Fistula, Anthracosis, silicosos, Infarct, Lung abscess.

B. Dissminated multiple pulmonary opacities (Miliary Mottling)

* Infections — Miliary TB, Bronchopneumonia, Brucellosis, Histoplasmosis, Coccidiodoconiosis, Blastomycosis.
* Inhalations — Pneumoconiosis, Berylliosis, Iodisted Oil (bronchochography), Mineral Oil (nose drops), Aspiration.
* Caridovascular — Heamosiderosis, Pulmonary Oedema, Multiple Pulmonary infarcts, Fat emboli.
* Allergic — Loeffer's syndrome, Asthma, Ascarasis.
* Bronchial — Excessive bronchiectesis, Mucoviscidosis.
* Neoplastic — Alveoler cell carcinoma of bronchus.
* Reticulosis — Lymphadenoma. Lymphoma, Leukaemia, Polycythemia.
* Others — Sarcoidosis, Rheumatoid arthriris, Hyaline membrane disease, Interstitial fibrosis, Honey-comb lung.

C. Causes of Hypertranslucency

Unilateral	*Bilateral*
Chestwall : Mastectomy, Polio, Scoliosis	* Diffuse obstructive emphysema.
Congenital : Absence of pectoral muscle	* Senile emphysema
Pulmonary : Emphysema artery hypoplasia	* Bronchial asthma
bullae : Main pulmonary artery hypoplasia	* Bullae
Pleura : Pneumothorax, contralateral pleural	* Bilateral Penumothorax
Effusion or pleural thickening	* Massive embolism
	* Primary pulmonary hypertension
	* Congential heart disease-Tetralogy of Fallot, Ebstein's anomaly, Pulmonary atresia.

D. Causes of Hilar Enlargement

Unilateral	*Bilateral*
* Tuberculosis	* Tuberculosis
* Bronchogenic carcinoma	* Sarcoidosis
* Metastatic adenopathy	* Fungal infection
* Sarcoidosis	* Lymphoma
* Fungal disease	* Pneumoconiosis
* Mediastinal masses	* Metastatic malignancy
* Lymphnode hyperplasia	* Erythema nodosum
* Others - Lymphatic leukaemia Pulmonary stenosis	* Others - Leukaemia acute massive pulmonary embolism

E. Causes of Cavitation in Chest

Cavity (containing air or fluid)	*Solid Mass within a cavity*
* Abscess	* Aspergillosis
* Bronchogenic carcinoma	* Blood clot in cavity
* Tuberculosis	* Breaking down neoplasm
* Mycotic cavitation	* Complicated hydatid cyst

F. Causes of Calcification inChest

- * Chest wall — Costal cartilages, Healing rib fractures, Tubercular glands, Cysticerci, breast tumour, Guinea worm, Osteomas, Chondromas
- * Tracheobronchi — Senile
- * Pleura — Plaques following T.B., Empyema, Pneumoconiosis, Hemothorax
- * Mediastinal — Lymphadenopathy (T.B., Sarcoid, Pneumoconiosis), Tumours (thyroid adenoma, aneurysm, dermoid cyst)
- * Lungs — Infections (T.B., Abscess , Fabrotic scars, Fungal infections), Vascular (hematoma, AV aneurysm), tumours (Hamartoma, Secondaries), Unknown (Broncholiths, Mitral stenosis)
- * Heart — Valves, Pericardium, Aortic arch (atherosclerosis, Syphilis), Left atrium (In MS), Coronary arteries, Patent ductus

G. Causes of Rib Notching

* Idiopathic
* Vascular — Coarctation of aorta, Taussig-Blalock operation, Obstructive arteritis, Pulmonary oligemia, (Pul monary stenosis, Fallot's Tetralogy, Ebstein's anomaly), Venous (SVC or IVC obstruction), A V fistulae
* Neurofibromatosis

H. Causes of Pulmonary Edema

Acute glomerulonephritis
Aspiration
Cardiac failure (left heart)
Drowning
Drug hypersensitivity
Drug overdose (heroin)
Fluid overload
High altitude
Intracranial disease
Malaria (falciparum)
Mediastinal tumor (with venous or lymphatic obstruction)
Oxygen toxicity
Shock lung
Uremia

I. Causes of Pulmonary Fibrosis-Diffuse

Chemical inhalation (late stage)
Dermatomyositis
Desquamative pneumonia
Hamman-Rich syndrome
Histiocytosis X
Idiopathic pulmonary hemosiderosis
Mucoviscidosis
Mycotic dieases
Neurofibromatosis
Pneumoconioses (organic and inorganic)
Radiation fibrosis
Rheumatiod lung
Sarcoidosis
Scleroderma
Tubercoulosis
Tuberous sclerosis

J. Causes of Kerely B Lines

Congestive failure
Diffuse intersitial fibrosis of varied etiology
Hamman-Rich sydndrome
Interstitial lower lobe pneumonia
Lipoid pneumonia
Lymphangitic metastases
Mitral stenosis
Pneumoconioses
Pulmonary alveolar proteinosis (unususal)
Sarcoidosis

K. Causes of Atelectasis (Obstructive)

Inflammatory	*Neoplastic*	*Other*
Middle lobe syndrome	Bronchial adenoma	Agammaglobulinemia
Pertussis	Bronchogenic carcinoma	Bronchial asthma
Tuberculosis	Invasive mediastinal	Chondromalacia of bronchus
		Foreign body
		Lymph node enlargement (peribronchial)
		Mucoviscidosis
		Papilloma of bronchus
		Peritoneal dialysis
		Postoperative mucus plug

L. Pneumothorax

Bronchopleural fistula
Bullous emphysema
Chemical pneumonitis
Histiocytosis X
Honeycomb lung
Ruptured esophagus
Spontaneous pneumothorax
Staphylococcal pneumonia
Trauma
Tuberculosis

M. Pleural Fluid and/or Thickening

Inflammatory	*Neoplastic*	*Other*
Amoebiasis	Bronchogenic carcinoma	Acute pancreatitis
Bacterial pneumonia	Hodgkin's disease	Asbestosis
Coccidiodomycosis	Leukemia	Cirrhosis
Coxsackie infections	Lymphosarcoma	Constrictive pericarditis
Empyema	Malignant mesothelioma	Familial Mediterranean fever
Hemophilus influenzae pneumonia	Metastatic disease	
Mycoplasma pneumonia	Primary macroglobulinemia of Waldenstrom	Heart failure
Nocardiosis		Lupus erythematosus
Pneumococcal pneumonia		Meigs's syndrome
Staphylococcal pneumonia		Nephrotic syndrome
Tularemia		Peritoneal dialysis
Tuberculosis		Postmyocardial infarction syndrome
Q fever		Pulmonary infarction
Viral pneumonia		Rheumatoid arthritis
		Subdiaphragmatic abscess
		Superior vena caval obstruction
		Trauma

O. Causes of Elevation of Diaphragm

Unilateral	*Bilateral*
* Eventration	* Infants
* Scoliosis	* Obesity
* Phrenic nerve palsy	* Ascites
* Avulsion or crush	* Pregnancy
* Basal pleural or Lung infection infarct	* Large abdominal mass
* Subphrenic infection	* Intestinal distention
* Subdiaphragmatic Tumor	* Large liver
	* Bilateral intrathoracic infection

ALVEOLAR DISEASE

Classic appearance of air space consolidation :

* Acinar rosettes : rounded poorly defined nodules in size of acini (6-10 mm). best seen at periphery of densities
* Air alveologram/bronchogram
* Butterfly/batswing distribution : peribilar
* Coalescent diffuse infiltrates with ill-defined borders
* Changes occur rapidly

CT :

* Poorly marginated densities within primary lobule (up to 1 cm in size)
* Rapid coalescence with neighbouring lesions in segmental distribution
* Predominantly central location with sparing of subpleural zones
* Air bronchograms

Diffuse air space disease

mnemonic : "*AIRSPACED*"

Aspiration

Inhalation

Renal

Swimming (drowning)

Pneumonia

Alveolra proteinosis

Cardiovascular

Edema

Drug reaction

CHRONIC ALVEOLAR INFILTRATE

mnemonic : " 1 DALLAS"
Inflammation (TB + fungus)
DIP (not consolidative)
Alveolar proteinosis
Lymphoma
Lipoid pneumonia
Alveolar cell carcinoma
Sarcoidosis

"STALLAG"
Sarcoidosis
Tuberculosis
Alveolar cell carcinoma
Lymphoma
Lipoid pneumonia
Alveolar proteinosis
Good pasture syndrome

SIGNS OF ACUTE INTERSTITIAL DISEASE

* Thickening of interlobular fissures
* Kerley-lines (=thickened connective septa)
* Kerley A line relatively long fine linear shadows in upper lungs, deep within lung parenchyma
* Kerley B lines=short horizontally oriented lines extending to pleura, perpendicular to pleura in costophrenic angles +retrosternal clear space
* Perironchial cuffing = thickened bronchial wall + peribonchial sheath (when viewed end on)
* Blurring of pulmonary vascular markings
* Increased density at lung bases
* Small pleural effusions

SIGNS OF CHRONIC INTERSTITIAL DISEASE

* Irregular visceral pleural surface
* **Reticulations** = network of interlacing lines
  (a) fine reticulations = early potentially reversible/minimal irreversible alveolar septal abnormality
  (b) coarse reticulations in 75% related to environmental disease, sarcoidosis, collagen-vascular disorders, chronic interstitial pneumonia
* **Nodularity**
  90% related to infectious/noninfectious granulomatous process, metastatic malignancy, pneumoconioses, amyloidosis
* **Linearity**
  Cardiogenic/noncardiogenic interstitial pulmonary edema, lymphangitic malignancy, diffuse bronchial wall disorders (cystic fibrosis, bronchiectasis, hypersensitivit asthma)
* **Honeycombing** = rounded radiolucencies< 1 cm in diameter set off against background of increased lung density (end stage lung) : "HIDE FACTS"
  Hamman-Rich, Hemosiderosis
  Infection, irradiation, Idiopathic
  Dust, Drugs

Eosinophillic granuloma, Edema
Fungal, Farmer's, lung
Aspiration (oil), Arthritis (rheumatoid, ankylosing spondylitis)
Collagen disease
Tumor, TBC, Tuberous sclerosis
Sarcoidosis, Scleroderma

HONEYCOMB LUNG

mnemonic : "HIPS RDS"
"B CHIPS"

Histiocytosis X
Bronchiectasis
Intersitital pneumonia
Pneumoconiosis
Collagen-vascular disease
Sarcoidosis Histiocytosis X
Intersitital pneumonia
Rheumatoid lung
Pneumoconiosis
Dermatomyositis
Sarcoidosis
Scleroderma

AIR-CRESCENT SIGN

1. Invastive pulmonary aspergillosis
2. Nonivasive mycetoma
3. Septic emboli
4. Cavitating benign + malignant neoplasma
5. Enchinococcal cyst
6. TB with Rasmussen anecurysms (most are too small to be identified on CXR)

BENIGN LUNG TUMOR

A. Central location
   1. Bronchial polyp
   2. Bronchial papilloma
   3. Granular cell myoblastoma
   = cell of origin from neural creast
   Age : middle-aged, esp, black women
   * endobronchial lesion in major bronchial

B. *Peripheral location*

1. Hamartoma
2. Leiomyoma benign metastasizing leiomyoma, Hx of pelvic surgery (hysterectomy)
3. Amyloid tumor not associated with amyloid of other organs/rheumatoid arthritis/myeloma
4. Intrapulmonary lymph node
5. Arteriovenous malformation
6. Endometrioma, Fibroma, neural tumor, Chemodectoma

C. *Central/Peripheral*

1. Lipoma (a) subpleural (b) endobronchial

D. *Pseudotumor*

1. Fibroxanthoma/Xanthogranuloma
2. Plasma cell granuloma
3. Sclerosing hemangioma middle-aged woman, RML/RLL (most commonly), may be multiple
4. Pseudolymphoma
5. Round atelectasis

MASS WITHIN CAVITY

1. Mycetoma = aspergilloma
2. Tissue fragment within carcinoma
3. Necrotic lung within abscess
4. Disintegrating hydatid cyst
5. Intracavitary blood clot

RADIOGRAPHIC SIGNS OF PNEUMOTHORAX IN SUPINE POSITION

1. *Anteromedial pneumothorax (earliest location)*
   * sharp delineation of mediastinal contours (SVC, azygos vein, left subclavian artery, anterior junction line, superior pulmonary vein, heart border, IVC, deep anterior cardiophrenic sulcus, pericardial fat pad)
   * outline of medial diaphragm under cardiac silhouette

2. *Subpulmonic pneumothorax* (second most common location)
   * hyperlucent upper abdominal quadrant
   * deep lateral costophrenic sulcus
   * visualization of anterior costophrenic sulcus
   * visualization of inferior surface of lung
   * sharply outlined diaphragm inspite of parenchymal disease
3. *Apicolateral pneumothorax (least* common location)
   * visualization of visceral pleural line
4. *Posteromedial pneumothorax* (in presence of lower lobe collapse)
   * lucent triangle with vertex at hilum
   * V-shaped base delineating costovertebral sulcus
5. Pneumothorax outlines pulmonary ligament

MEDIASTINAL MASS

(excluding hyperplastic glands, granuloma, lymphoma metastases)

1. Neurologenic tumors (28%) : malignant in 16%
2. Teratoid lesion (19%) : malignant in 15%
3. Enterogenous cyst (16%)
4. Thymomas (13%) : malignant in 46%
5. Pericardial cysts (7%)
   * 75% of all mediastinal tumors are benign (in all age groups)
   * 1/3 diagnosed on routine chest X-ray
   * 2/3 found in association with symptoms (pain, cough, shortness of breath)
   * 80% of malignant tumors are symptomatic

Anterior mediastinal mass

mnemonic : **"4 Ts"**

Thymoma

Teratoma

Thyroid tumor/goitre

Terrible lymphoma

A. *Solid Thymic Lesions*
   1. Thymoma (benign, malignant); most common
   2. Normal thymus (neonate)

3. Thymic hyperplasia (child)
4. Thymolipoma
5. Lymphoma

B. *Solid Teratoid Lesions*

1. Teratoma
2. Embryonal cell carcinoma
3. Choriocarcinoma
4. Seminoma

C. *Thyroid/Parathyroid*

1. Substernal thyroid/goiter
2. Thyroid adenoma/carcinoma
3. Ectopic parathyroid adenoma ectopia in 10% (62% in anterior mediastinum, 30% within thyroid tissue.

   8% in posterior superior mediastinum)

D. *Lymph Nodes*

1. Lymphoma (Hodgkin, NHL) : may arise in thymus, more common in young adults
2. Metastases
3. Benign lymph node hyperplasia
4. Angioblastic lymph adenopathy
5. Mediastinal lymphadenitis : Sarcoidosis/granulomatous infection

E. *Cardiovascular*

1. Tortuous brachiocephalic artery
2. Aneurysm of ascending aorta
3. Aneurysm of Sinus of Valsalva
4. Dilated SVC
5. Cardiac tumor
6. Epicardial fat pad

F. *Cysts*

1. Cystic hygroma
2. Bronchogenic cyst
3. Extralobar sequestration
4. Thymic cysts/Dermoid cysts
5. Pericardial cyst :
   (i) true cyst
   (ii) Pericardial diverticulum
6. Pancreatic pseudocyst

G. *Others*

1. Neural tumor (vagus, phrenic, lipoma)
2. Paraganglioma
3. Hemangioma/Lymphangioma
4. Mesenchymal tumor (fibroma, lipoma)
5. Sternal tumors
   (a) Metastases from breast, bronchus, kidney, thryoid
   (b) Malignant primary (chondrosarcoma, myeloma, lymphoma)
   c) Benign primary (chondroma, aneurysmal bone cyst, giant cell tumor)
6. Primary lung/pleural tumor (invading mediastinum)
7. Mediastinal lipomatosis :
   (a) Cushing disease
   (b) Corticosteroid therapy
8. Morgagni hernia/Localized eventration
9. Abscess

Middle mediastinal mass

A. *Lymph Nodes*

90% of masses in the middle mediastinum are malignant

(a) Neoplastic Adenopathy
   1. Lymphoma (Hodgin : NHL = .1)
   2. Leukemia (n 25%) : lymphocytic > granulocytic
   3. Metastasis (bronchus, lung, upper GI, prostate, kidney)
   4. Angioimmunoblatic lymphadenopathy

(b) Inflammatory Adenopathy
   1. Tuberculosis/Histoplasmosis (may lead to fibrosing mediastinitis)
   2. Blastomycosis (rare)/Coccidioidomycosis
   3. Sarcoidosis (predominant involvement of paratracheal nodes)
   4. Viral pneumonia (particularly measles + Cat Scratch fever)
   5. Infectious mononucleosis/Pertussis pneumonia
   6. Amyloidosis
   7. Plague/Tularemia
   8. Drug reaction
   9. Giant lymph node hyperplasia = Castleman disease
   10. Connective tissue disease (rheumatoid, SLE)
   11. Bacterial lung abscess

(c) Inhalational Diseases Adenopathy
   1. Silicosis (eggshell calcification, also in sarcoidosis + tuberculosis)
   2. Coal-worker's pneumoconiosis
   3. Berylliosis

B. *Foregut Duplication Cysts*
   1. Bronchogenic/respiratory cyst (cartilage, respiratory epithelium)
   2. Enteric cyst
   3. Extralobar sequestration (anomalous feeding vessel)
   4. Hiatal hernia

C. *Primary Tumors (infrequent)*
   1. Carcinoma of trachea
   2. Bronchogenic carcinoma
   3. Esophageal tumor : leiomyoma, carcinoma, leiomyosarcoma
   4. Mesothelioma
   5. Granular cell myoblastoma of trachea (rare)

D. *Vascular lesions*
   1. Aneurysm
   2. Distended veins (SVC, azygos vein)
   3. Hematoma

Posterior mediastinal mass

A. *Neoplasm*
   1. Ganglion series tumors (in children)
      * 80% are elongated with tapered borders
      1. Neuroblastoma : highly malignant undifferentiated small round cell tumor originating in sympathetic ganglia, < 10 years of age
      2. Ganglioneuroma : benign tumor from mature ganglion cells.
      3. Ganglioneuroblastoma : both features, spontaneous maturation possible
   (b) Nerve root tumors (in adults)
      * 80% appear as round masses with sulcus
      1. Schwannoma : derived from sheath of Schwann without nerve cells
      2. Neurofibroma : contains Schwann Cells + nerve cells, 3 + 4 th decade
      3. Malignant schwannoma

(c) Paraganglioma (rare)
1. Chemodectoma
2. Pheochromocytoma
* rib spreading, erosion, destruction
* enlargement of neural foramina (dumb-bell lesion)
* scalloping of posterior aspect of vertebral body
* scoliosis

CT : * low density soft tissue mass ('lipid contents)

2. Spine tumor : Metastases (e.g. bronchogenic carcinoma), ABC, chondrosarcoma, Ewing sarcoma
3. Lymphoma
4. Invasive thymoma
5. Mesenchymal tumor (Fibroma, Lipoma, Leiomyoma)
6. Hemangioma
7. Lymphangioma
8. Thyroid tumor

B. Inflammation
1. Paraspinous abscess (tuberculosis)
   * destruction of endplates + disc space
2. Mediastinitis
3. Lymphoid hyperplasia
4. Sarcoidosis (in 2%, typically asymptomatic patient)
5. Pancreatic pseudocyst

C. Vascular Mass
1. Aneurysm of descending aorta (curvillinear calcification ; elderly)
2. Enlarged azygos + accessory hemiazygos vein
3. Esophageal varices

D. Trauma
1. Traumatic aneurysm/Pseudoaneurysm
2. Hematoma
3. Loculated hemothorax
4. Traumatic pseudomeningocele

E. Congenital
* Cysts may demonstrate peripheral rimi-like calcifications
1. Enteric cyst
2. Neurenteric cyst (hemi/-butterfly vertebra)
3. Bronchogenic cyst
4. Extralobar sequestration

F. Other
1. Loculated pleural effusion
2. Bochdalek hernia
3. Pancreatic pseudocyst
4. Lateral meningocele (neurofibromatosis; enlarged neural foramen)
5. Lipoma/lipomatosis
6. Extramedullary hematopoiesis (in chronic bone marrow deficiency) paraspinal area rich in RES-elements
   * splenomegaly; widening of ribs
7. "Pseudomass" of the newborn
8. Teratoma (rare)

ENLARGEMENT OF AZYGOS VEIN

A. Collateral circulation
1. Portal hypertension
2. SVC obstruction
3. IVC obstruction
4. Azygos continuation of IVC

B. Heart Disease
1. Right heart failure
2. Constrictive pericarditis
3. Pericardial effusion

EGG SHELL CALCIFICATION OF NODES

A. Pneumoconiosis
1. Silicosis (5%)
2. Coal worker's pneumoconiosis (1.3-6%) not seen in; asbestosis, berylliosis, talcosis, baritosis

B. Sarcoidosis (5%)

C. Fungal + bacterial infection (rare).
1. Tuberculosis
2. Histoplasmosis
3. Coccidiodomycosis

D. Lymphoma following radiation therapy

RIGHT CARDIOPHRENIC ANGLE MASS

1. Epicardial fat pad/lipoma (*most common* cause)
   * triangular opacity in cardiophrenic angle less dense than heart
   * increase under corticosteroid treatment
2. Pericardial cyst
3. Aneurysm
4. Dialated right atrium
5. Diaphragmatic hernia
6. Diaphragmatic lymph node (esp. in Hodgkin disease + breast cancer)
7. Primary lung mass
8. Anterior mediastinal mass

UNILATERAL PLEURAL EFFUSION

1. Neoplasm
2. Infection (TB)
3. Collagen vascular disease
4. Subdiaphragmatic disease
5. Pulmonary emboli
6. Trauma
7. Chylothorax

LEFT-SIDED PLEURAL EFFUSION

1. Spontaneous rupture of the esophagus
2. Dissecting aneurysm of the aorta
3. Traumatic rupture of aorta distal to left subclavian artery
4. Transection of distal thoracic duct
5. Pancreatitis : left sided (68%), right-sided (10%), bilateral (22%)
6. Pancreatic + gastric neoplasm

RIGHT -SIDED PLEURAL EFFUSION

1. Congestive heart failure
2. Transection of proximal thoracic duct
3. Pancreatitis

PLEURAL SOLITARY MASS

= density with incomplete border and tapered superior + inferior borders, difficult to distinguish from chest wall mass (rib destruction *reliable).*

1. Loculated pleural effusion (*"vanishing tumor")*
2. Organized empyema
3. Metastasis
4. Local benign mesothelioma
5. Subpleural lipoma; may erode adjacent rib
6. Hematoma
7. Mesothelial cyst
8. Neural tumor (schwannoma, neurofibroma)
9. Fibrin bodies : 3-4 cm tumorlike concentrations of fibrin forming in serofibrinous pleural effusions; usually near lung base.

MULTIPLE PLEURAL DENSITIES

* Diffuse pleural thickening with lobulated borders

1. Loculated pleural effusion :
   infectious, hemorrhagic, neoplastic
2. Metastasis (most common cause) :
   predominantyly adenocarcinoma
3. Diffuse malignant mesothelioma
   almost always unilateral, associated with asbestos exposure
4. Malignant thymoma (rare)
   * contiguous speread, invasion of pleura, spreads aroud lung
   * No pleural effusion
5. Thoracic aplenosis

= autotransplantation of splenic tissue to pleural sac following thoracic abdominal trauma; discovered 10-30 years later

* Positive Tc-99m sulfur colloid scan

PLEURAL CALCIFICTAION

A. *Trauma*

1. Healed hemothorax = Fibrothorax :
   * Hx of significiant chest trauma
   * healed rib fracture
2. Radiation therapy

B. *Infaction*

1. Healed empyema
2. Tuberculosis (and RX for TB: pneumothorax/oleothorax), histoplasmosis

C. *Pneumoconiosis*

1. Asbestos-related pleural disease (most common):
   * combination of basilar reticular interstitial disease (<1/3) + pleural thickening
   * Calcifications of parietal pleura frequentely diagnostic (diaphragmatic surface of pleura, bilateral but asymmetric)
2. Talcosis : similar to asbestos-related disease
3. Bakelite
4. Muscovite mica

D. *Hypercalcemia*

1. Pancreatitis
2. Secondary hyperparathyroidism renal failure/scleroderma

E. *Miscellaneous*

1. Mineral oil aspiration
2. Pulmonary infarction

mmemonic : "TAFT"

Tuberculosis

Asbestosis

Fluid (effusion, empyema, hematoma)

Talc

DIAPHRAGM

Bilateral diapharagmatic elevation

A. Shallow inspiration (most frequent)

B. Abdominal causes

1. Obesity 2. Pregnancy 3. Ascities 4. Largé abdominal mass

C. Pulmonary causes

1. Bilateral atelectasis
2. Restrictive pulmonary disease (SLE)

D. Neuromuscular disease

1. Myasthenia gravis
2. Amyotrophic lateral sclerosis

Unilateral diaphragmatic elevation

1. Subpulmonic pleural effusion
   * dome of diaphragm migrates towards the costophrenic angle and flattens
2. Altered pulmonary volume
   (a) Atelectasis
      * associated pulmonary density
   (b) Postoperative lobecomy/pneumextomy
      * rib defects, metallic sutures
   (c) Hypoplastic lung
      * Small hemithorax (more often on the right), crowding of ribs, mediastinal shift, absent/ small pulmoanry artery, frequently associated with dextrocardia + anomalous pulmonary venous return
3. Phrenic nerve paralysis
   (a) Primary lung tumor
   (b) Malignant mediastinal tumor
   (c) Iatrogenic
   (d) Idiopathic
      * Paradoxic motion on fluoroscopy (patient in lateral position sniffing)
4. Abdominal disease

(a) Subphrenic abscess : history of surgery, acompanied by pleural effusion

(b) Distended stomatch/colon

(c) Interposition of colon

(d) Liver mass (tumor, echinococcal cyst, abscess)

5. Diaphragmatic hernia
6. Eventration of diaphargm
7. Traumatic reputure of diaphargm
8. Diaphragmatic tumor

mesothelioma, fibroma, lipoma, lymphoma metastases

MALIGNANT TUMORS OF CHEST WALL IN CHILDREN

1. Ewing Sarcoma of rib (most common)

(a) Older child : rib involvement in 7%, predominant involvement of pelvis + lower ectermity

(b) Child < 10 years : rib involvement in 30%

2. Rhabdomyosarcoma

relatively common in children + adolescents

* Sclerosis/destruction/scalloping of cortex (local extention to contigious bone)
* may calcify

Matastases to : lung, ocasionally lymph nodes

prognosis : infiltrative growth with high risk of local recurrence

3. Neuroblastoma

10% percent as chest wall mass

4. Asking tumor

= uncommon tumor probably arising from intercostal nerves in young Caucasian females

Path : neurobalstoma small cell tumor containing neuron-specific enolase (may also be found in neuroblastoma)

* rib destruction
* pleural effusion

Metastases to : bone, CNS, liver, adrenal

PNEUMONIA

"Classic" pneumonia pattern

1.	Lobar distribution	:	Streptococcus pneuromoniae
2.	Bulging fissure	:	Klebsiella
3.	Pneumatocele	:	Staphyococcus
4.	Pulmonary edema	:	Viral pneumonia, Pneumocystic pneumonia
5.	Alveolar nodules	:	Varicella, bronchogenic spread of TB

Lobar pneumonia

= Alveolar pneumonia

= pathogens reach peripheral air space, incite, exudation of watery edema into alveolar space, centrifugal speread via small airways, pores of Kohn + Lambert into adjunct lobules + Segments

* Nonsegmental sublobar consolidation
* Round pneumonia (= uniform involvement of contiguous alveoli)
  (a) Streptococcus pneumoniae
  (b) Klebsiella pneumoniae (more aggressive); in immunocompromised + alcholics
  (c) Any pneumonia in children
  (d) Atypical measles
* Expension of lobe with bulging of fissures
* Lung necrosis with cavitation

  DDx : aspiration, pulonary embolus

Lobular penumonia

= Bronchopneumonia

= Inflammatory response in conducting airways + surrounding parenchyma

* Small fluffy ill - defined nodules which enlarge with time
* Lobar + segmental densities with volume loss from airway obstruction secondery to bronchial narrowing + mucus plugging

  Organisms :

  Pseudomonas, Klebsiella penumoniae, Bacillus proteus, E, coli, Anaerobes (Bacteroides + Clostridia), Legionnares bacillus, Staphylococcus aureus, Nocardiosis, Actinomycosis

Actue Interstitial penumonia

Inititally predominantly affecting interstitial tissues

Organisms : Virues, mycoplasma. Pneumocystic

* Often subacute atypical pneumonia
* Diffuse interstitial process with peribronchial thickening
* segmentl/lobar densities (mucus pluging + damage of surfactant producing type 2 alveolar cells)

Cavitating pneumonia

1. Staphylococcus aureus
2. Haemophilus influenzae
3. S. pneumonia

other Gram-negative organisms (e.g. Klebisella)

Cavitating opportunistic infections

A. Fungal infections
   1. Aspergillosis
   2. Nocardiosis
   3. Mucormycosis (= phycomycosis)

B. Septic Emboli
   1. Anaerobic organisms

C. Staphylococcal Absecess

D. TuberculosisNummmular from

Repeated infections insame paitent are not necessarily due to same organism!

DDx : 1. Metastatic disease in carcinoma/Hodgkin disease

RECURRENT PNEUMONIA IN CHILDHOOD

A. *Immune problem*
   1. Immune problem
   2. Chronic granulomatous disease of childhood (males)
   3. Alpha 1- antitrypsin deficency

B. *Aspiraton*
   1. Gastroesophageal reflux
   2. H-type trachesophageal fistula
   3. Disorder of swallowing mechanism
   4. Esophageal obstruction, impacted esophageal forign body

C. *Underlaying lung disease*

1. Sequestration
2. Bronchopulmonary dysplasia
3. Cystic fibrosis
4. Atopic asthma
5. Bronchiolitis obliterans
6. Sinusitis
7. Bronchiectasis
8. Ciliary dysmolities syndromes
9. Pulmonary foreign body

DRUG-INDUCED PULMONARY DAMAGE

A. *Chemotherapeutic*

1. Busulfan = Myelarn (for CML)

   dose-dependent toxicity after 3-4 years on the drug in 1 - 10%

   * Diffuse linear pattern (occasionally reticulonodular/nodular pattern)
   * Partial/complete clearing after withdrawal of drug

     DDx : penumocystis pneumonia, interstitial leukemic infiltrate

2. Bleomycin (for squamous cell carcinoma, lymphoma, testicular tumor)

   Toxicity at doses > 300mg (in 3 - 6%);

   increased toxicity with age + radiation therapy + high oxygen concentrations

   * Subpleural linear/nodular opacities in lower lung zones occuring after 1- 3 months following begining of therapy

3. Nitrosoureas = BCNU, CCNU (for glioma, lymphoma, myeloma)

   Incidence of 50% after doses > 1500mg/sqm

   * Linear finely nodular opacities (following treatment of 2 -3 years)
   * High incidence of pneumothorax

4. Methotrexate, procarbazine (for AML, psoriasis, pemphigus)

   Not dose-related, usually self-limited despite continuation of therapy

   * Blood eosinophilia (common)
   * Linear/reticulonodular process (time delay of 12 days to 5 days to 5 years, usually early)
   * acinar filling pattern (later)
   * transient hilar adenopathy + pleural effusion (on occasion)

     DDX : pneumo cystis pneumonia

B. *Nitrofurantoin*

(a) Acute disorder wiht fever + eosinophilia (Commonest presentation)

(b) Chronic reaction with interstitial fibrosis(less common), may not be associated with peripheral Eosinophilia

* Positive for ANA + LE cells
* prompt resolution after withdrawal from drug

C. *Heroin, propoxypheme, Methadone*

Overdose followed by pulmonary edema in 30 - 40 %

* Bilateral widespread air space consolidation
* Aspiration pneumonia in 50 - 75 %

D. *Salicylates*

* Asthma
* Pulmonary edema(with chronic ingestion)

E. *Intravenous contrast agent*

* Pulmonary edema

F. *Amiodarone (for refractory ventriculatory arrhythmia)*

* Pulmonary insufficiency after 1-12 months in 14 - 18 % on long term therapy
* Alveolar + Interstitial infiltrates
* Peripheral consolidation
* pleural thickening adjacent to consolidation .

METASTASES TO LUNG

Pulmonary metastases occur in 30% of all malignancies; mostly hematogenous

Age : > 50 years (in 87%)

Frequency :

	Origin of pulmonary metastasis		*Probability of pulmonary metastasis*	
1.	Breast	22%	Kidney	75%
2.	Kidney	11%	Osteosarcoma	75%
3.	Head and Neck	10%	Choriocarcinoma	75%
4.	Colorectal	9%	Thyroid	65%
5.	Uterus	6%	Melanoma	60%
6.	Pancreas	5%	Breast	55%
7.	Ovary	5%	Prostate	40%
8.	Prostate	4%	Head and Neck	30%
9.	Stomach	4%	Esophagus	20%

Incidence of pulmonary metastases :
menmonic "CHEST"

Choriocarcinoma	60%
Hypernephroma/Wilms tumor	30/20%
Ewing sarcoma	18%
Sarcoma (osteo-/-rhabdomyosarcoma)	15/21%
Testicular tumor	12%

* Multiple nodules (in 75%) of varying sizes (most typical), 82% subpleural
* Cavitated nodules (4%)
  (75% are squamous cell carcinomas from head and neck + GU system)
* Calcified nodules (<1%) : osteo and chondrosarcoma, papillary carcinoma of thyroid, ovarian carcinoma, lung metastases following radiation/chemotherapy
* Fine micronodular pattern : highly vascular tumor (renal cell, breast, thyroid, prostate carcinoma, bone sarcoma, choriocarcinoma)
* Pneumothorax (2%): especially in children with bone tumors

CT :

* Noncalcified multiple (>10) round lesions > 2.5 cm likely to be metastatic
* Connection to pulmonary arterial branches

CALCIFYING METASTASES

mnemonic : ***"BOTTOM"***

Breast
Osteosarcoma
Thyroid
Testicular
Ovarian
Mucinous adenocarcinoma

* PULMONARY ARTERY CONFIGURATION

Large (convex) pulmonary artery

Pulmonary valve stenosis

Left-to-right shunts

Cardiac admixture lesions

Pulmonary hypertension

Pulmonary insufficiency

Hypoplastic left heart (neonate)

Interrupted aortic arch (infant)

Infantile coarctation aorta (infant)

Idiopathic dilation (adolescent)

post-tetralogy of Fallot repair

Aneurysm

Absent pulmonary Valve

* SMALL (CONCAVE OR FLAT) PULMONARY ARTERY

Infundibur Pulmonary stenosis (tetralogy of Fallot)

Hypoplastic right heart syndrome (neonate)

Ebstein's anomaly

Transposition of great vessels

Truncus arteriosus

* UNEQUAL PULMONARY ARTERY BRNACHES

Tetralogy of Fallot

Truncus arteriosus

Hypoplastic pulmonary artery and lung

Acquired hypoplastic lung (Swyar-james)

Pulmonary Valve stenosis (in childhood)

Unilateral pulmonary vein atresia

Hemitruncus arteriosus

ORIGINAL SOLVED MCQ's IN DM PULMONARY MEDICINE

1. **Following are characteristics of restrictive lung disease, except :**
   A. Reduction in all lung volumes
   B. Increase in all lung volumes
   C. Rapid shallow breathing
   D. Alveolar hyperventilation
2. **The most important contributing factor for the development of corpulmonale in chronic bronchitis is :**
   A. Hypoxia B. Hypercapnia
   C. Acidosis D. Alkalosis
3. **Features of lipid pneumonia can include following, except :**
   A. Paraffinoma B. Mineral oil ingestion
   C. Fat laden macrophages D. Hilar adenopathy
4. **Clinical features of massive pulmonary embolism include all of the following except :**
   A. Breathlessness and syncope
   B. Central and peripheral cyanosis
   C. Elevated jugular venous pressure and heart rate
   D. Pleuritic chest pain and haemoptysis
5. **The following are contributing factors to the development of chronic bronchitis and emphysema :**
   A. α-1-antitrypsin deficiency
   B. Chronic respiratory infections
   C. Cigarette smoking
   D. All of the above
6. **Which one is incorrect for malignant pleural effusion :**
   A. Transudate in character
   B. Stony dull percussion note
   C. Haemorrhagic fluid
   D. Causes severe dyspnoea
7. **Primary atypical pneumonia is caused by a :**
   A. Myocoplasma B. Fungus
   C. Bacteria D. Spirochaete
8. **Cyanosis and clubbing are early coexisting features in :**
   A. Lung abscess

Ans.	1. B	2. A	3. D	4. B	5. D	6. A
	7. A	8. B				

B. Fibrosing alveolitis
C. Bronchogenic carcinoma
D. Chronic bronchitis

9. **Bronchoalveolar lavage is beneficial in the evaluation of :**
A. Interstitial lung disease B. Acute bronchitis
C. Bronchopleural fistula D. Pneumothorax

10. **Respiratory failure is diagnosed by :**
A. Deterioration in exercise tolerance
B. Tachypnoea and cyanosis
C. Arterial blood gas analysis
D. Pulmonary spirometric analysis

11. **Monday dyspnoea is seen in :**
A. Byssinosis B. Pulmonary eosinophilia
C. Malingering D. Chronic bronchitis

12. **Sudden bout of cough, followed by catch in breath and increasing dyspnoea indicates the diagnosis of :**
A. Pleural effusion B. Myocardial infarction
C. Pneumothorax D. Lobar pneumonia

13. **Pulmonary infiltrates with eosinophilia are seen in all of the following except :**
A. Bronchial asthma B. Ascaris infestation
C. Malaria D. Polyarteritis

14. **Adult respiratory distress syndrome is observed in following except :**
A. Falciparum malaria B. Snake bite
C. Status asthmaticus D. Toxic shock syndrome

15. **Consider the following statements about hypersensitivity pneumonitis :**
1. Precipitins can be demonstrated in the serum
2. Lung parenchyma shows granulomatous inflammation
3. Environmental agents are involved
4. Skin tests are negative

Of these statements
A. 1 and 4 are correct B. 1,3 and 4 are correct
C. 1,2 and 3 are correct D. 2,3 and 4 are correct

16. **Alveolar hypoventilation is observed in :**
A. Guillain-Barre syndrome B. Status asthmaticus
C. Bronchiectasis D. Chronic bronchitis

Ans.	9. A	10. C	11. A	12. C	13. C	14. C
	15. B	16. A				

17. **Mycoplasma infection simulates :**
   A. Pneumococcal pneumonia
   B. Viral pneumonia
   C. Hypersensitivity pneumonia
   D. Aspiration pneumonia

18. **A patient with pulmoanry tubeculosis is infection :**
   A. Till sputum AFB is negative
   B. Till culture negativity is confirmed
   C. Till radiological cavity disappears
   D. In the initial few weeks after optimal exposure of drugs

19. **Which of the following statements about pulmonary embolism is false ?**
   A. It is associated with prolonged bed rest
   B. Most emboli arise from clots in the right ventricle
   C. It has a known association with femoral fracture
   D. It may cause sudden death

20. **Fibreoptic bronchoscopy is preferred for :**
   A. Endobronchial biopsy
   B. Massive haemoptysis
   C. Bronchoalveolar lavage
   D. All of the above

21. **A patient with clubbing and bilateral crackles in lower lobes has :**
   A. Consolidation B. Bilateral bronchiectasis
   C. Interstitial lung disease D. Bronchiolitis

22. **Commonest cause of respiratory failure type I is :**
   A. Pleural effusion
   B. Chronic bronchitis with emphysema
   C. Bronchiectasis
   D. Aspergillosis

W23. **Upper respiratory tract infections are common in :**
   A. Tetralogy of Fallot B. Cystic fibrosis
   C. Mitral Regurgitation D. Waegner's granulomatosis

24. **Treatment of Bronchial asthma include following except :**
   A. Breathing exercises
   B. Inhalational steroids
   C. Inhalational theophylline
   D. Prophylactic B2 agonists

25. **Haemoptysis with Renal involvement is seen in :**
   A. Good pasture's syndrome B. Rheumatoid arthritis
   C. Reiter's disease D. Behcet's disease

Ans.	17. B	18. D	19. B	20. D	21. C	22. B
	23. B,D	24. C	25. A			

26. In Tuberculosis in an AIDS patient, the Chest X-ray looks like :
A. Millary shadow
B. Cavity
C. Consolidation
D. Collapse

27. Late response in Bronchial asthma is because of :
A. Mast cells
B. Neutrophils
C. Macrophages
D. Eosinophils

28. Not true about acute bronchopulmonary asperigillosis :
A. Pleural effusion
B. Centrilobar atelectasis
C. Lungs main involvement
D. Involves diseased lungs

29. Aspirin sensitive asthma is associated with :
A. Extrinsic asthma
B. Urticaria
C. Nasal polyp
D. Obesity

30. Staphylococcal pneumonia, following are true except :
A. Lobar destruction
B. Pneumatocele formation
C. Hilar lymphadenopathy
D. Resistant to treatment

31. Following are features of Pancoast tumor except :
A. Excessive sweating
B. Miosis
C. Ptosis
D. Loss of ciliospinal reflex

32. Which type of CA lung commonly causes Horner's Syndrome :
A. Squamous cell CA
B. Oat cell CA
C. Adenocarcinoma
D. None of the above

33. Following conditions are associated with Asbestosis except :
A. Mesotheliom
B. Pleural thickening
C. Lung cancer
D. Bronchiectasis

34. Legionnaire's penumonia can present with :
A. Bilateral infiltrates
B. Dry cough
C. Diarrhoea
D. All of the above

35. Bilateral mottling of lung is :
A. Miliary Tuberculosis
B. Varicella pneumonia
C. Both
D. None

36. Following are true about Acute bronchial asthma except :
A. Cyanosis
B. Monosyllabilic speech
C. Decreased respiratory rate
D. Intercostal muscle retraction

37. Increased resistance to airflow during expiration is due to :
A. High vapour saturation
B. Compression of airways
C. Turbulent flow of air
D. Bronchoconstriction

Ans.	26. A	27. D	28. A	29. C	30. C	31. A
	32. A	33. D	34. D	35. C	36. C	37. B

38. Clubbing is seen in except :
A. Cirrhosis B. Emphyema
C. Left to right shunt D. Pulmonary A.V. fistula

39. Acute epiglottitis is most commonly caused by :
A. Herpes simplex B. Haemophilus influenza
C. Group B streptococcus D. Klebsiella

40. Bronchial asthma is associated with raised levels of :
A. PGI2 B. PGH2
C. Leuktrienes D. Thromboxane

41. Smoking is associated with following malignancies except :
A. Bladder B. Kidney
C. Liver D. Pancreas

42. Exudative pleural effusion is seen in following except :
A. Cirrhosis B. Rheumatoid arthritis
C. Dressler's syndrome D. Lymphoma

43. Chronic respiratory failure is caused by following except :
A. ARDS B. Chronic bronchitis
C. Emphysema D. Bronchiectasis

44. Investigation of choice in Bronchiectasis is :
A. X-ray B. Bronchoscopy
C. Bronchography D. Ultrasound

45. Lung abscess is not a complication of :
A. Bronchiectasis B. Lobar pneumonia
C. Bronchopneumonia D. Malignancy

46. The confounding factor in mesothelioma caused by Asbestosis is :
A. Smoking B. Alcoholism
C. Tuberculosis D. Rheumatoid arthritis

47. Treatment of choice in Pneumocystis carinii pneumonia is :
A. Co-trimoxazole B. Pentamidine
C. Ciprofloxacin D. Ziduvidine

48. One of the following is not seen with controlled ventilation :
A. Baro trauma B. Alkalosis
C. Pulmonary embolism D. Cardiac tamponade

49. All of the following are poor prognostic indicators in acute severe asthma except :
A. pCO2-60 mmHg B. pO2-30 mm Hg
C. pH-7.5 D. Pulsus paradoxus

50. Following are associated with unilateral pulmonary edema except :
A. Pneumoconiosis B. Aspiration pneumonitis
C. Lymphoma D. Post pleural aspiration

Ans.	38. C	39. B	40. C	41. C	42. A	43. A	44. C
	45. C	46. A	47. A	48. D	49. C	50. A	

51. **Functional residual capacity is measured by following :**
A. Deep inspiration
B. Forceful expiration
C. Normal expiration
D. Shallow inspiration

52. **The commonest presenting symptoms of bronchial adenoma is :**
A. Haemoptysis
B. Dyspnoea on sitting up
C. Cough
D. Chest pain

53. **Not a complication of chronic bronchitis :**
A. Amyloidosis
B. Emphysema
C. Spontaneous pneumothorax
D. Cor pulmonale

54. **Pancoast's tumor : True statement is :**
A. Affects left lower lobe
B. Causes radicular pain in upper limb
C. Produces recurrent laryngeal N. palsy
D. Cerebral psudotumour

55. **A 40-year old patient with a history of having been treated for pulmonary tuberculosis 10 years back presents with weight loss and recurrent haemoptysis of six months duration. His sputum of AFB is repeatedly negative. His X-ray chest shows a cavitatory lesion in the right upper lobe with an ill defined cavity within it. The most appropriate line of management will be :**
A. Surgical resection
B. Antitubercular drugs
C. Antifungal drugs
D. Broad spectrum antibiotics

56. **Increased neutrophil count in bronchoalveolar lavage fluid is characteristic of :**
A. Sarcoidosis
B. Hypersenstivity pneumonitis
C. Fibrosing alveolitis
D. Miliary tuberculosis

57. **Which one of the following therapies would be safe in patient with pulmonary tuberculosis having markedly abnormal liver function ?**
A. Streptomycin+isoniazid
B. Ethambutol+isoniazid
C. Rifampicin+isoniazid
D. Streptomycin+Ethambutol

58. **A 17-year old boy with thalassemia major has been admitted with a history of fever and respiratory distress of 10 days duration. His respiratory rate is 36/minute, arterial PO2 is 40 mm Hg. and PCO2 is 30 mm Hg. His chest X-ray shows bilateral basal infiltration. The most likely diagnosis is :**
A. Pneumococcal pneumonia
B. Mycoplasma pneumonia
C. Pneumocystis carinii pneumonia
D. Miliary tuberculosis

Ans.	51. C	52. A	53. A	54. B	55. A	56. C
	57. D	58. C				

59. All of the following are true of 'multi-drug resistant' tuberculosis except :
A. It is caused by mycobacteria other than M. tuberculosis
B. It is treated by a combination of 4 to 6 drugs
C. Surgical treatment, wherever feasible is preferred
D. It is common in patients with Acquired Immunodeficiency Syndrome (AIDS)

60. The differential diagnosis of pulmonary embolism includes all but :
A. Costochondritis
B. Pancreatitis
C. Perforated peptic ulcer
D. Lung abscess

61. Massive hemoptysis with pneumonia with multiple cavitites in lung is seen in :
A. Good Pasture syndrome
B. Ca. Bronchus
C. Wegener's granulomatosis
D. Chronic Bronchitis

62. If FEV1=1.3 lit, FVC, = 3.1 lit, in an adult male, the pattern is suggestive of :
A. Normal lung function
B. Restrictive lung disease
C. Obstructive lung disease
D. None of the above

63. For diagnosis of respiratory failure blood gas study should show :
A. PaCO2-40 mm Hg
B. PaCO2-5 mm Hg
C. PaCO2-more than 50 mm Hg and PaO2 less than 50 mm Hg
D. PaCO2-30 mm Hg
E. PaCO2-120 mm Hg

64. Pneumatocele is commonest in :
A. Pneumococcal Pneumonia
B. Staphylococcal Pneumonia
C. H. Influenzae Pneumonia
D. Viral Pneumonia

65. Expiratory wheeze is produced due to :
A. Blockage of larger air passages
B. Blockage of smaller air passages
C. Bronchiectasis
D. Lobar pneumonia

66. The most common type of bronchogenic carcinoma is :
A. Epidermoid
B. Anaplastic
C. Alveolar
D. Transitional

67. Decreased FEV1 and increased Tidal volume is seen in :
A. Emphysema
B. COAD
C. Br. asthma
D. TB

Ans.	59. B	60. D	61. C	62. C	63. C	64. B
	65. B	66. A	67. A			

68. Which of the following statements about the respiratory physiology of the normal adult at rest is false ?

A. The alveolar ventilation is approximately 5 litres per minute
B. The pulmonary blood flow is approximately 10 litres per minute
C. The arterial carbon dioxide tension is in the range of 35-45 mmHg
D. The oxygen consumption is about 250 ml/minute

69. Exercise induced asthma :

A. Seen only in extrinsic asthmatics
B. Seen more in swimmers than runners
C. Induced by cold air exposure
D. Allergy induced

70. Features of fat emoblism occurs in :

A. < 6 hours
B. 6-12 hours
C. 12-24 hours
D. 24-72 hours

71. Causes of COPD does not include :

A. Chr. bronchitis
B. Br. Asthma
C. Mitral stenosis
D. Interstitial pulm. disease

72. A pleural tumour associated with clubbing and arthralgia is :

A. Hamartoma
B. Carcinoid
C. Fibrom
D. Mesothelioma

73. In a case of extrinsic asthma, precipitating factors include all of the following except :

A. Exposure to antigen
B. Excitement
C. Infection & irritants
D. Salt ingestion

74. About psittacosis, one of the following is true :

A. Bacterial aetiology
B. Secondary infections are common
C. Haemolytic anaemia
D. Responds to tetracycline
E. Severe tracheitis

75. Features of cryptogenic fibrosing alveolitis include except :

A. Reduced FVC
B. Clubbing
C. Crepitations in the lower and mid zones
D. Peripheral cyanosis

76. The oxygen content of the arterial blood is reduced in all of the following except :

A. Methaemoglobinaemia
B. Carbon monoxie poisoning
C. By the presence of a left to right shunt in the heart
D. Fallot's tetralogy
E. Fibrosing alveolitis with low arterial $PaCO_2$

Ans.	68. B	69. C	70. D	71. C	72. D	73. D
	74. D	75. D	76. C			

77. **Causes of a blood stained pleural effusion include :**
A. Pulmonary tuberculosis B. Pulmonary embolism
C. Ca lung D. All of the above

78. **Exudate pleural effusion is found in the following conditions except :**
A. Meig's syndrome B. Malignancy
C. Pulmonary infarction D. Tuberculosis

79. **In bronchial asthma, there is constriction of :**
A. Large airway B. Medium airway
C. Terminal bronchiole D. Respiratory bronchiole

80. **True about idiopathic fibrosing alveolitis is :**
A. ↓ Total lung capacity B. ↑ Residiul volume
C. ↓ FeV1/FEV D. ↓ Forced expiratory volume

81. **Tropical eosinophilia is manifested as :**
A. Nocturnal asthma
B. Detected on peripheral blood smear evaluation
C. Segmental consolidation
D. Any of the above

82. **Paradoxical breathing is characteristic of :**
A. Pneumonia B. Pneumothorax
C. Atelectasis D. Diaphragmatic paralysis

83. **Stony dull note on percussion is characteristic of :**
A. Pleural effusion B. Consolidation
C. Pleurisy D. Tuberculosis cavity

84. **Tubular breathing is seen in :**
A. Pleural effusion B. Consolidation
C. Pleurisy D. Tuberculous cavity

85. **Cavenous breathing is seen in :**
A. Pleural effusion B. Consolidation
C. Pleurisy D. Tuberculous cavity

86. **Commonest cause of spontaneous pneumorthax is :**
A. Rupture of sub-pleural bleb
B. TB
C. Trauma
D. Asthma

87. **Volume of air taken into the lungs in normal respiration is known as :**
A. Vital capacity B. Timed vital capacity
C. Tidal volume D. Inspiratory reserve volume

Ans.	77. D	78. C	79. C	80. A	81. D	82. D
	83. A	84. B	85. D	86. A	87. C	

88. A 50-year-old patient previously in good health and sudden onset of right anterior chest pain without chills, fever or cough. On physical examination, he was tachypneic and had a temperature of 99.4F. Over the right lower rib cage there was an inspiratory rub. Chest X-ray was negative. Which statement is correct.

A. Viral pneumonia is the most likely diagnosis
B. Pneumococcal pneumonia is most likely and penicillin should be given
C. Pulmonary embolus must be considered promptly
D. Bronchoscopy needs to be done promptly
E. Bronchogenic carcinoma is most likely

89. Hyperventillation may lead to :

A. Tetany
B. Respiratory acidosis
C. Metabolic acidosis
D. Metabolic alkalosis

90. About pulmonary embolism, all are true except :

A. Dysponea
B. Severe chest pain
C. Hypoxaemia
D. Normal PO2

91. In chronic obstructive pulmonary disease, bronchoconstriction is caused by all except :

A. Cold air inhalation
B. Disodium cromoglycate
C. Asbestos inhalation
D. Smoking

92. Localized wheezing in seen in :

A. Lobar pneumonia
B. Foreign body in lung
C. Atelectesis
D. Pulmonary abscess

93. Ominous sign in bronchial asthma is :

A. Cyanosis
B. Feeble breath sounds and absent wheezing
C. Pulsus paradoxus
D. Accessory muscles functioning

94. Aspergillosis is not seen with :

A. Tuberculosis
B. Silicotuberculosis
C. Sarcoidosis
D. Malignant cavity

95. To achieve plurodesmosis in a malignant pleural effusion, the drug used in :

A. Polymyxin B
B. Chloromycetin
C. 1% betadine
D. Tetracycline

96. Negative Mantoux test is important in :

A. Pulmonary Koch's
B. Sarcoidosis
C. Carcinoma bronchus
D. Lymphoma

Ans.	88. C	89. A	90. D	91. B	92. B	93. B
	94. C	95. D	96. A			

97. Ethambutol induced optic nerve toxicity :

A. Dose related B. Not dose related
C. Caused by prolonged use D. None of the above

98. Hormone producing carcinoma bronchus manifests :

A. Hormonal changes earlier than other changes
B. Hormonal changes after other changes
C. Simultaneously
D. During remission

99. In miliary tuberculosis, findings may be :

A. Thrombocytopenia B. Leucopenia
C. Myelofibrosis D. All of the above

100. Tuberculosis is reactivated in :

A. Pregnancy B. Steroid therapy
C. Malnutrition D. All of the above

101. A young cultivator has been admitted with sudden onset of cough and severe dyspnoea Physical examinations reveals central cyanosis, tachycardia and basal crackles. The most likely diagnosis is :

A. Acute severe asthma
B. Left ventricular failure
C. Hypersensitivity pneumonitis
D. Pulmonary embolism

102. Best view to diagnosis minimal pleural effusion is :

A. PA B. Supine AP
C. Oblique D. Lateral decubitus

103. Tuberculosis in adults :

A. Has adenopathy B. Is low infectious
C. Is less symptomatic D. Is localized

104. Triad seen in Carcinoma lung include following except :

A. ↑ ADH B. ↑ ACTH
C. ↑ Calcium levels D. ↑ Growth hormone

105. In inflammatory exudate, true is :

A. Protein contents is 3-8 gm/dl
B. Cell count less than 5/cmm
C. Specific gravity 1001
D. All of the above

106. Obstructing hemithorax is seen in :

A. Pneumothorax B. Massive pleural effusion
C. Consolidation D. Atelectesis

Ans. 97. A 98. A 99. D 100. D 101. C 102. D
103. D 104. D 105. A 106. D

107. Hyperpnoea in exercise is because of :

A. Hypercapnia
B. Hypoxaemia
C. Reflex
D. Stimulation of cortex and proprioceptors

108. At rest, ventillation is drived by :

A. O2 B. CO2
C. pH D. HCO3

109. The technique of "chromosomal walking" has been especially utilized to locate gene of :

A. Emphysema
B. Hyaline membrane disease
C. Cystic fibrosis
D. Pulmonary Histiocytosis X

110. To produce air embolism minimum air required is :

A. 50 ml B. 100 ml
C. 150 ml D. 200 ml

111. Safe oxygen concentration in oxygen therapy should be :

A. 2% B. 20%
C. 33% D. 37%

112. Status asthmaticus is nowdays known as :

A. Malignant Asthma B. Non responsive Asthma
C. Episodic Asthma D. Severe Acute Asthma

113. Commonest cause of death in sarcoidosis is :

A. Pneumonia B. Cor pulmonale
C. Myocardial infarction D. Liver failure

114. The following about Klebsiella pneumonia are true except :

A. Red current jelly sputum
B. Seen in alcoholics
C. Seen in older age group
D. Penicillin is the drug of choice

115. Eaton Lambert syndrome is seen with :

A. Oat cell carcinoma B. Myasthenia gravis
C. Thyroid cancer D. Pancreatic head cancer

116. A 43 year old man begins to wheeze. There is no way to tell whether this is bronchial asthma or cardiac asthma. The best drug to use would be :

A. Digitalis B. Aminophylline
C. Epinephrine D. Cortisone

Ans.	107. D	108. B	109. C	110. B	111. C	112. D
	113. D	114. D	115. A	116. B		

117. A positive tuberculin test includes :
A. Strong immunity
B. Tuberculous infection
C. Disseminated tuberculosis
D. Primary complex

118. The pathognomonic physical sign of tuberculous cavity in the lung is :
A. Bronchial breath sound B. Whispering pectoriloquy
C. Puerile breathing D. Posttussive suction

119. Miliary tuberculosis is caused by :
A. Haematogenous spread from a primary focus
B. Bronchogenic spread
C. Contiguity from a tuberculous focus
D. Reactivation of healed focus

120. Chemoprophylaxis in T.B. in given to :
A. Uniinfected persons
B. Tuberculosis
C. Extrapulmonary tuberculosis
D. Treatment of failure cases

121. Tension Pneumothorax occurs in :
A. Open pneumothorax
B. Clossed pneumothorax
C. Valvular pneumothorax
D. Oesophageal rupture

122. Hamman's sign is positive in ———emphysema :
A. Mediastinal B. Surgical
C. Panacinar D. Interstitial

123. A 30 year old man after an accident is conscious. Next day, he develops dyspnoea and X-ray chest shows perihilar lymphadenopathy, Correct diagnosis is :
A. Aspiration pneumonia B. Embolism
C. Myocardial infarction D. Cardiac temponade

124. Which of the following is not a feature of Kartagener syndrome :
A. Bronchiectasis B. Pancreatic insufficiency
C. Sinusitis D. Situs inversus

125. Frothy pink sputum is seen in :
A. Bronchogenic carcinoma B. Collapse lung
C. Actinomycosis lung D. Pulmonary oedema

Ans.	**117. B**	**118. D**	**119. A**	**120. A**	**121. C**	**122. A**
	123. A	**124. B**	**125. D**			

126. After 2 weeks of the treatment of infectious tuberculosis, the efficiency of therapy is indicated by :

A. Reduced ESR
B. Weight gaining
C. Skiagram improvement
D. Reduction tubercule bacilli in smear

127. Which of the following is the commonest causative agent of bacterial pneumonia in childhood :

A. Streptococcus haemolyticus group A
B. Streptococcus haemolyticus group B
C. Streptococcus pneumoniae
D. Esch. coli
E. Haemophilus inflenzae B

128. Whispering pectoriloquy is seen in :

A. Collpase of peripheral bronchus
B. Pneumonia
C. Bronchitis
D. All of the above

129. Pulmonary haemosiderosis may be associated with :

A. Myocarditis
B. Collagen disease
C. Glomerulonephritis
D. Mitral stenosis
E. All of the above

130. True about bronchoalveolar carcinoma :

A. Common in smokers
B. Seen usually in asbestosis
C. Sensitive to radiotherapy
D. Multifocal in origin

131. In severe pulmonary emphysema, pulmonary arterial pressure is :

A. Elavated
B. Decreased
C. Elevated only in the presence of pulmonary arteriosclerosis
D. Decreased only in presence of corpulmonale

132. Rifampicin should be used with appropriate caution when the following drug is prescribed :

A. Oral contraceptives
B. Corticosteroids
C. Digoxin
D. All of the above drugs

133. Principal phagocytes in the lung are :

A. Megakaryocytes
B. Alveolar macrophages
C. Lymphocytes
D. Neutrophils

134. Which of the following antitubercular drug can be best used in patients with hepatic dysfunction :

A. Streptomycin
B. INH
C. Ethambutol
D. Thiacetazone

Ans.	126. D	127. C	128. B	129. E	130. A	131. A
	132. D	133. B	134. A			

135. **Following exposure to the tubercle bacillus the amount of time necessary by the tuberculin skin test to the positive is :**
A. 2-4 weeks
B. 4-6 weeks
C. 3 months
D. 6 months
E. 1 year

136. **Least common tumour of the pleura is :**
A. Fibroma
B. Haemangioma
C. Mesothelioma
D. Metastasis

137. **Which of the following is the best parameter of ventilation :**
A. Blood pH
B. Forced expiratory volume (FEV)
C. Blood PCO2
D. Blood PO2
E. Vital capacity

138. **Which type of Emphysema is caused by smoking :**
A. Central
B. Lobular
C. Paraseptal
D. Panacinar

139. **There is no correlation between X-ray findings & clinical features of :**
A. Mycoplasma pneumonia
B. Friedlander's pneumonia
C. Pneumococcal pneumonia
D. Staphylococcal pneumonia

140. **Shrinking lung syndrome is seen in :**
A. SLE
B. Systemic sclerosis
C. Polymyositis
D. Dermatomyositis

141. **In which type of hypoxia oxygen is given ?**
A. Hypoxic hypoxia
B. Histotoxic hypoxia
C. Stagnant hypoxia
D. Anaemic hypoxia

142. **Management of spontaneous pneumothorax with only slight retraction of lung and minimal symptoms should be :**
A. Thoracic pump
B. Multiple needle aspirations
C. Observation
D. Single needle aspiration

143. **Pyopneumothorax is most likely to ensue following a pneumothorax in which of the following cases :**
A. Silicosis
B. Sarcoidosis
C. Lung abscess
D. Normal individual

144. **Hypercapnoea at rest is most indicative of :**
A. Hypoventilation
B. Right to left shunt
C. Impaired diffusion
D. CO poisoning

145. **Closed needle biopsy of the lung is contraindicated in :**
A. Tuberculosis
B. Pulmonary hypertension
C. Hamartoma
D. Suspected carcinoma

Ans.	135. B	136. B	137. C	138. D	139. B	140. A
	141. A	142. C	143. C	144. A	145. B	

146. DLCO measurement is increased in following except :

A. Emphysema
B. Fresh haemorrhage in Good Pasture syndrome
C. Respiratory sarcoidosis
D. Interstitial lung disease

147. Excessive mucus production in the bronchial tree and expectoration of sputum best describes :

A. Chronic bronchitis
B. Acute pneumonia
C. Asthma
D. Emphysema

148. Chest tightness towards the end of first day of work week (Monday chest tightness) is due to :

A. Bagassosis
B. Bysinosis
C. Silicosis
D. Coal dust

149. An agricultural worker that develops acute dyspnoea with chills, fever and cough in the presence of hay, may have :

A. Bagassosis
B. Hay fever
C. Allergic interstitial pneumonitis
D. Fungal pneumonia

150. Bowing of fissures is seen in :

A. Pneumococcal Pneumonia
B. Klebsiella Pneumonia
C. Staphylococcal Pneumonia
D. Mycoplasma Pneumonia

151. Dilatation of large bronchi with destruction of bronchial wall is seen in :

A. Asthma
B. Bullae
C. Emphysema
D. Bronchiectasis

152. Characteristically in pulmonary tuberculosis :

A. Involvement of posterior portion of upper lobe
B. Wheezing never seen
C. Pleura never seen
D. Foul sputum

153. Characteristically the primary focus of tuberculosis in lung usually includes the following except :

A. Usually near pleura
B. Spread to local lymph nodes
C. Initialy exudative
D. Non caseation

154. Pulmonary embolism without infarction can be suspected on chest X-ray by all, except :

A. Atelectatic streaks
B. Abrupt cutt off vessel
C. Large pleural effusion
D. Relatively normal X-ray

Ans.					
146. B	147. A	148. B	149. C	150. D	151. D
152. A	153. D	154. C			

155. Bronchial asthma patient on artificial ventilation requires :

A. A low inspiratory flow

B. An equal I.E. ratio of 1 : 1

C. An inverse ratio ventilation

D. An I.E ratio 1 : 2.5

156. Which of the following is not associated with obstructive pulmonary emphysema ?

A. Hypercapnoea B. Secondary polycythaemia

C. Respiratory alkalosis D. Peptic ulcer

157. Fine creptiations maximal at the end of inspiration are characteristic of :

A. Byssinosis B. Bronchiectasis

C. Pulmonary oedema D. Fibrosing alveolitis

E. α-antitrypsin deficiency

158. Which is incorrect about Friedlander's pneumonia ?

A. Rare

B. Rapidly fatal

C. Massive consolidation and excavation of one or more lobes

D. Chocolate brown sputum

E. Lower lobe is usually involved

159. Most early feature of Bronchial carcinoma is :

A. Cough B. Haemoptysis

C. Pain chest D. Dyspnoea

E. Anorexia and loss of the weight

160. Endemic haemoptysis is caused by :

A. Paragonimus westermani B. Fasciolopsis buski

C. Schistosomia haematobiu D. Clonorchis sinensis

161. The pathology in primary pulmonary hypertension is associated with all of the following except :

A. Internal hyperplasia

B. Muscular hypertrophy of media

C. Plexiform vascular lesions

D. Thrombosis in larger pulmonary vessels

162. Most common cause of non inflammatory fluid in the pleural cavity is :

A. Neoplasm B. Nephrosis

C. Cirrhosis D. Congestive heart failure

Ans.	155. D	156. C	157. D	158. E	159. A	160. A
	161. D	162. D				

163. A bloody pericardial effusion may be due to :

A. Tumor involving the pericardium
B. Tuberculous pericarditis
C. Uraemic pericarditis
D. All of the above

164. In acute asthmatic attack :

A. Subcutaneous adrenaline is the treatment of choice
B. Chest is held in inspiration
C. Oxygenation is contraindicated
D. Hydrocortisone cures it immediately

165. The commonest cause of massive haemoptysis is :

A. Lobar pneumonia
B. Bronchiectesis
C. Tuberculosis
D. Lung abscess

166. A boy of 18 has a moderately severe attack of asthma. One would expect to find :

A. PO2 less than 60 mmHg (8.0 kPa)
B. PCO2 greater than 60 mmHg (8.0kPa)
C. Raised plasma bicarbonate
D. Immediate relief by intravenous injection of hydrocortisone

W167. An exacerbation of Farmer's lung :

A. Is commoner in summer
B. Is characterised by intense wheeze
C. Produces eosinophilia in the peripheral blood
D. Is excluded by the absence of precipitating antibodies

168. Paraoxysmal nocturnal dyspnoea is common in :

A. Fallot's tetralogy
B. Pulmonary stenosis
C. Mitral stenosis
D. A.S.D.

169. Steroid inhalation side effect is :

A. Cushing syndrome
B. Oropharyngeal Candidiasis
C. Sedation
D. None

170. Sudden onset of cough followed by increasing dyspnoea is characteristic of :

A. Pleural effusion
B. Lobar pneumonia
C. Myocardial infarction
D. Pneumothorax

171. Drug of choice for exercise induced asthma :

A. Terbutaline
B. Ipratropium
C. Salbutamol
D. Sodium cromoglycate

Ans.					
	163. D	164. A	165. B	166. A	167. NONE
	168. C	169. B	170. D	171. B	

172. The most common cause of massive pleural effusion in a young female in our country is likely to be :

A. Adenocarcinoma of the bronchus
B. Secondaries in the pleura from adenocarcinoma of the ovary
C. Tuberculosis
D. Pneumonia
E. Systemic lupus erythematosus

173. Hemoptysis due to Rasmussen aneurysm occurs in :

A. Tuberculosis B. Sarcodosis
C. A V fistula D. Asbestos inhalation

174. In massive pulmonary embolism, the embolus may obstruct :

A. Rt. ventricular output B. Left ventricular output
C. Sup vena cava D. Pulmonary veins

175. A patient suffering from lung abscess develops anasarca. The probable reason is :

A. Amyloidosis B. Good Pasture syndrome
C. Pyelonephriti D. Acute renal failure

176. Schistosomiasis may be seen clinically presenting with :

A. Fever and allergic manifestation
B. Abdominal pain and diarrhoea
C. Cor pulmonale
D. All of the above

177. The principal indications for resection in pulmonary tuberculosis are all of the following except :

A. Persistence of cavity and excretion of bacilli
B. Emphyema
C. Need for a positive diagnosis
D. Persistence of bacilli in the sputum in a patient with a localised lesion
E. Bleeding associated with tuberculous bronchiectasis

178. Analgesic which can be safely used in a patient of aspirin induced asthma is :

A. Acetaminophen B. Piroxicam
C. Ibuprofen D. Indomethacin

179. All of the following are characteristic signs of cor pulmonale, except :

A. Hepatomegaly
B. Left parasternal heave
C. Immidiate blowing diastolic pulmonary murmur
D. Quiet P2

Ans.	172. C	173. A	174. D	175. A	176. D	177. B
	178. D	179. D				

180. PEEP (positive end expiratory pressures) known to result in following except :

A. Increased cardiac output

B. Opening of collapsed airways and reduction of intrapulmonary shunt

C. Pneumomediastinum

D. Tension pneumothorax

181. Which is incorrect of the following statement :

A. Smoking and chronic infection reduces mucociliary clearance

B. Reduced mucociliary clearance is specific for immotile cilia syndrome

C. Normal or slightly reduced mucociliary clearance rules out immotile cilia syndrome

D. The presence of immotile sperm is highly suggestive of and consistent with immotile cilial syndrome

182. Ultra structural abnormalities reported in defective cilial immotile cilia syndrome are :

A. Dynein arm deficiency

B. Absence of radial spokes

C. Absence of central microtubule

D. All of the above

183. Investigation of choice to distinguish between COPD with emphysema and bronchial asthma is :

A. Allergy test to pollens B. Methacholine provocation test

C. Chest X-ray D. Arterial blood gas analysis

184. With alpha 1 antitrypsin (AAT) deficiency all are true except :

A. Small proportion of deficient individual encounter major problems in early life

B. Development of lung disease can be modified by avoidance of cigarette smoking and use of AAT injection

C. The risk to develop liver disease is high for women

D. The development of liver disease shows a strong intrafamilial correlation

185. Of the following, the feature that most clearly separates the emphysematous from the bronchitis patient with chronic, irreversible obstructive airway disease :

A. Residual volume elevation

B. Hyperinflation on chest radiograph

C. Arterial oxygen tension at rest

D. Static lung compliance and lung recoil pressure

Ans.	180. A	181. B	182. D	183. A	184. C	185. D

186. Essential steps in the management of massive life threatening hemoptysis include all of the following except :

A. Emergency bronchoscopy to localize the site of bleeding
B. Notification of thoracic surgeon
C. Maintaining the affected lung in non-dependant position
D. Immediate chest radiography

187. For diagnosis of obstructive airway diseases, which of the following measurement is useful :

A. Vital capcity
B. Timed vital capcity
C. Tidal volume
D. Blood gas analysis

188. Sudden bout of cough, followed by catch in breath and increasing dyspnoea, indicates the diagnosis of :

A. Pleural effusion
B. Pneumothorax
C. Myocardial infarction
D. Lobar pneumonia

189. Controlled oxygen therapy is given in :

A. Cyanotic heart disease
B. Acute pulmonary oedema
C. Bronchial asthma
D. Chronic corpulnonale with respiratory failure

190. Which of the extrapulmonary site is most frequently involved by tuberculosis :

A. Pericardium
B. Peritoneum
C. Spine
D. Testes

191. Persons living at high altitude are more prone to develop which of the following chronic illness :

A. Pulmonary edema
B. Pulmonary hypertension
C. Emphysema
D. Kyphoscoliosis

192. Recurrent aspiration pneumonia is caused by :

A. Dermatomyostis/Polymyositis
B. Rheumatoid arthritis
C. Progressive systemic sclerosis
D. Systemic lupus erythromatosis

193. Remittent fever, cyanosis and thick purulent sputum which reveals numerous cocci clustered within the leukocytes on Gram staining, the most probabale diagnosis is :

A. Pneumococcal pneumonia
B. Klebsieela pneumonia
C. Streptococcal pneumonia
D. Staphylococcal pneumonia

Ans.	186. C	187. B	188. B	189. D	190. C	191. B
	192. C	193. D				

194. Muscle of expiration is :

A. Diaphragm B. Internal intercostal
C. External intercostal D. Rectus abdominis

195. Respiratory symptoms are associated with :

A. Rocky Mountain spotted fever
B. Strongyloidiasis
C. T. solium
D. Onchocerca

196. A patient has aspergillosis (moving ball) in a tubercular cavity. The most likely presenting feature is :

A. Recurrent hemoptysis
B. Allergic bronchopulmonary aspergillosis
C. Pulmonary eosinophilia
D. Acute pneumonia

197. Increased alveolar PA02-Pa02 is seen in :

A. Poliomyelitis
B. Fibrothorax
C. Primary alveolar hypoventilation syndrome
D. Interstitial disease

198. Which of the following is not true about bronchiectasis :

A. Increased incidence in rheumatoid arthritis
B. Streptococcus most common organism causing infection
C. Long term antibiolic coverage required
D. Clubbing is usually present

199. Cor pulmonale is rarely caused by :

A. Pectus excavatum (funnel chest)
B. Pulmonary tuberculosis
C. Obstructive emphysema
D. Sarcoidosis

200. Patient with stab injury in left 5th intercostal space in mid clavicular line, an examination showed pulse 140/min BP 120/80 mmHg, RR 20/min. Clinical examination revealed trachea in midline, distal heart sounds and normal air entry on both sides. Most likely diagnosis is :

A. Dissection of thoracic aorta
B. Pneumothorax
C. Cardiac temponade
D. Haemopneumothorax

201. Longterm complication of bronchopulmonary dysplasia is :

A. ↓ FRC B. Small airway disease
C. Large airway disease D. Interstitial lung disease

Ans.	194. D	195. B	196. A	197. D	198. C	199. A
	200. C	201. B				

202. Hypertrophic pulmonary osteoarthropathy is characterized by :

A. Lack of pain even in the presence of advanced changes
B. Development only in the presence of clubbed digits
C. Primarilly proximal involvement of the long bones
D. All of the above
E. None of the above

203. Which of the following is most likely to be associated with bronchiectasis of the main bronchi :

A. Allergic bronchopulmonary aspergillosis
B. Endobronchial tuberculosis
C. Measles
D. Chronic bronchitis

204. Respiratory failure type I consists of :

A. Low PaO_2, normal or low $PaCO_2$
B. Raised $PaCO_2$, low PaO_2
C. PaO_2, $PaCO_2$ - low
D. PaO_2 & $PaCO_2$ - high

205. Not a known cause of ARDS :

A. Nitrofurantoin B. CCF
C. Chlorine gas D. Amniotic fluid embolism

206. All are true of adult respiratory distress syndrome (ARDS), except :

A. The typical morphology is necrotizing fibrinous bronchpneumonia
B. Type alveolar cells are destroyed early in the disease process
C. Severe arterial hypoxaemia refractory to O_2 therapy
D. An immunologic pathogenetic pathway has been propounded in some cases
E. None of these

207. A malignant lymphoma characterized by a higher incidence in women, propensity for involvement of mediastinal and supraclavicular lymph nodes, and the presence of lacunar cells is most likely to be :

A. Hodgkin's lymphoma, mixed cellularity type
B. Hodgkin's lymphoma, nodular sclerosis type
C. Hodgkin's lymphoma, lymphocytic predominance
D. Hodgkin's lymphoma, lymphocytic depleted
E. N.H.L. undifferentiated type

208. Allergic aspergillosis, all are true except :

A. Bronchial asthma B. Central bronchiectesis
C. Parenchymal infiltration D. Pleural effusion

Ans.	202. B	203. A	204. B	205. B	206. A	207. B
	208. D					

209. Cough is a recognized sideeffect of :

A. Cyclosporine
B. Hydrallazine
C. Encainide
D. Lisinopril
E. Nifedipine

210. A 60 year old man presents with H/o fever, chills, dry cough and a 15 minute rigors, suddenly developed right pleuritic chest pain, chest X ray revealed right middle lobe consolidation and blood smear showed leucocytosis with multiple band forms. Which of the following statements regarding pneumonia is correct :
Manipal 1998

A. If sputum examination shows gram positive diplo-cocci and pus cells, Empiric treatment with penicillin is sufficient
B. A negative blood culture would rule out the diagnosis of infecting organism
C. Absence of rigors excludes a diagnosis of pneumococcal pneumonia
D. All of the above

211. Colonization of pseudomonas on the respiratory epithelium is seen in :

A. Congenital cyst of lung
B. Cystic bronchiectasis
C. Cystic fibrosis of pancrea
D. Hydatid cyst

212. Pulmonary infiltration with peripheral eosinophilia syndrome is observed in all except :

A. Tropical eosinophilia
B. Polyarteritis nodosa
C. Ascariasis
D. Eosinophilic granuloma

213. Atelectasis may result from :

A. Neoplasm
B. Pneumothorax
C. Pulmonary embolism
D. Acute bronchitis
E. All of the above

214. Hypoxaemia while receiving 100% O2 indicates :

A. Impaired diffusion
B. Hypoventilation
C. Ventilation perfusion ratio inequality
D. Right to left shunt

215. Factors that suggest a need for admission to the hospital of a 24-year-old female having an asthmatic attack include :

A. Arterial Pa O2 of 68 mmHg
B. Hb of 15 gm/dl
C. Tachycardia of 116 beats/minutes
D. Eosinophilia

Ans.	209. D	210. A	211. C	212. D	213. E	214. D
	215. A					

216. Increased alveolar ventilation is characteristic of all the following clinical conditions, except for one :

A. Lactic acidosis B. Hepatic failure
C. Acute airway obstruction D. Pulmonary embolus

217. Respiratory depression may be produced by :

A. Trimethaphan B. Polymyxins
C. Aminoglycosides D. All of the above

218. The coughing in chronic bronchitis :

A. Cause waking in mid-night
B. May produce seizures
C. Cause worsening of dyspnoea
D. Cause worsening on change of posture

219. The least common cause of recurrent pneumonia is :

A. Cystic fibrosis
B. Tuberculosis
C. Past H/O traumatic spontaneous pneumothorax
D. Whooping cough in childhood

220. Which of the following is not seen in Ca bronchus :

A. Acanthosis nigricans
B. Hyperkeratosis of fingers and toes
C. Myositis
D. Nephrotic syndrome

221. All are true of chronic cor pulmonale except :

A. Prominent pulmonary segment
B. Dilated main pulmonary artery
C. Peripheral pruning of pulmonary artery
D. Kerley B lines

222. All predispose to ARDS except :

A. Fat embolism B. Septicemia
C. Multiple blood transfusio D. Status asthmaticus

223. Commonest cause of non-progressive pneumothorax is :

A. Rupture of subpleural bleb
B. Tuberculosis
C. Trauma
D. Bronchiectasis

224. Acute respiratory failure does not occur with :

A. Porphyria B. Myaesthenia gravis
C. Polio D. Pb poisoning

225. Alveolar-arterial tension gradient increases in following except :

A. Diffusion defects B. Hypoventilation
C. R—> L shunt D. Ventilation perfusion defect

Ans.	216. C	217. D	218. C	219. C	220. B	221. D
	222. D	223. A	224. D	225. B		

226. A patient with blood chemistry of pH 7.3, PCO2-65 mm, PO2 < 40 mm. Diagnosis is :

A. COPD
B. ARDS (Acute Resp. Distress Syndrome)
C. TOF (Tetralogy of Fallot)
D. None of the above

227. In case of COPD with corpulmonale, following are true except :

A. Respiratory failure always present
B. Cardiac output may be raised
C. Increased erythropoitin levels
D. Increased pulmonary wedge arterial pressure

228. Consider the following drugs :

1. Beclamethasone
2. Ipratropium bromide
3. Salbutamol
4. Nedocromil sodium

Those which are useful in reducing bronchial airway inflammation in asthma would include :

A. 1 and 2
B. 2 and 3
C. 3 and 4
D. 1 and 4

229. Corticosteroids are useful in status asthmaticus primarily because :

A. They are potent directly bronchodilator
B. They mimic dilator neurotransmitters
C. They antagonise the released mediators
D. They bring about a non specific reduction in inflammatory response

230. Curschmann's spirals in sputum are seen in :

A. Tuberculous cavity
B. Asthma
C. Bronchitis
D. Bronchiectasis

231. Commonest cause of bronchopleural fistula is :

A. Carcinoma bronchus
B. Bronchiectasis
C. Pulmonary TB
D. Bronchitis

232. Nasal congestion may be produced by following except :

A. Guanethidine
B. Reserpine
C. Isoproterenol
D. Levodopa

233. Air embolism is diagnosed by :

A. Loud P2
B. Continous murmur
C. Water wheel sound
D. Cresendo descresendo murmur

234. The commonest type of bronchopneumonia is :

A. Pneumococcus
B. Staphylococcus
C. Klebsiella
D. Aspiration type

Ans. **226. A** **227. D** **228. D** **229. D** **230. B** **231. C** **232. D** **233. C** **234. D**

235. In interstitial lung disease, following decrease except :

A. FVC
B. Compliance
C. Diffusion capacity
D. Alveolar to capacity gradient

236. The following results were obtained on arterial blood gas analysis in a 58-year old male (while breathing room air), hospitalised on account of increasing breathlessness :

pCO_2 = 76 mm Hg; pO_2 = 32 mmHg, pH = 7.34

The most likely diagnosis is :

A. Bronchial asthma
B. Interstitial lung disease
C. Chronic obstructive airway disease
D. Left ventricular failure

237. A middle-aged patient presents with a short history of high fever and rigors. On examination, the pulse rate is 140/min and there are signs of toxaemia. Chest examination shows restriction of movement over left infraclavicular region and there is dullness on percussion. Vocal resonance is increased with lowpitched bronchial breath sounds over the above area. The most likely diagnosis is :

A. Bronchial carcinoma
B. Lung abscess
C. Lobar pneumonia
D. Pleural effusion

238. The most common danger of fibre optic bronchoscopy is :

A. Hypoxaemia
B. Hypercapnia
C. Respiratory acidosis
D. Low arteriolar CO_2

239. Maximum midexpiratory flow in a female is ——— litres per sec :

A. 1.0
B. 1.6
C. 2.0
D. 3.0

240. Which of the following aerosol does not lead to broncho-constriction :

A. Water
B. Saline
C. Cold air
D. All of the above

241. Apnoea after hyperventilation is due to :

A. $\downarrow CO_2$
B. $\uparrow O_2$
C. $\uparrow CO_2$
D. $\downarrow O_2$

242. Obstructive sleep apnoea may result in all of the following except :

A. Systemic hypertension
B. Pulmonary hypertension
C. Cardiac arrhythmia
D. Duodenal ulcer
D. None of the above

Ans. 235. D 236. A 237. C 238. A 239. C 240. B
241. D 242. D

243. Decreased diffusion capacity is seen in the following except :
A. Emphysema
B. Pulm. vascular disease
C. Interstitial lung disease
D. Intracardiac shunt

244. Diffusing capacity for carbon monoxide (single breath) is ——— mL CO/min/mmHg :
A. 10
B. 25
C. 60
D. 75

245. Static recoil pressure at total lung capacity is ——— (±5 cm) H2O :
A. 10
B. 25
C. 50
D. 75

246. Hyperventilation is not associated with :
A. Chronic respiratory acidosis
B. Normal muscle effort
C. Normal lung
D. Hysteria

247. Cheyne Strokes breathing occurs when there is :
A. Varying pO2 and fixed CO2
B. Fixed pCO2 and pO2
C. Fixed pO2 and varying pCO2
D. Varying pO2 and pCO2

248. Unresolved fever after treatment of pneumonia is due to :
A. Collapse of lung
B. Empyema thoracic
C. Pneumothorax
D. Pulmonary embolism

249. Commonest cause of hydropneumothorax in our country is :
A. Bronchogenic carcinoma
B. Sarcoidosis
C. Emphysematous bulla
D. Pulmonary tuberculosis

250. All show wide Alveolar-Arterial O2 gradient except :
A. Bronchiectasis
B. ARDS (Acute Respiratory Distress Syndrome)
C. Interstitial fibrosis
D. Central hypoventilation

251. Multiple cavitary lesions of lungs are found in following except :
A. Pulmonary metastasis
B. Staph. pneumonia
C. Bronchiectasis
D. Cystic fibrosis

252. Cause of pulmonary fibrosis include following except :
A. Busulphan therapy
B. α-1 Antitrypsin deficiency
C. Chronic lead poisoning
D. Ankylosing spondylosis

253. Anti-tuberculous drug is be avoided in pregnant female is :
A. INH
B. Rifampicin
C. Pyrazinamide
D. Ethambutol

Ans.						
	243. D	244. B	245. B	246. B	247. D	248. B
	249. C	250. D	251. A	252. C	253. B	

254. The most sensitive and vulnerable tissue to oxygen lack in human beings is :

A. Heart B. Kidney
C. Liver D. Brain

255. Which of the following is not a cause of bronchial obstruction :

A. Radiation B. Sarcoidosis
C. Aspergillosis D. Cryptogenic fibrosis

256. Oxygen therapy is not much useful in

A. Hyaline membrane disease
B. Carbon monoxide poisoning
C. Left ventricular failure
D. Methhemoglobinemia

257. Which of the following is not true about bronchiectesis :

A. Increased incidence in rheumatoid arthritis
B. Streptococcus is the most common organism causing infection
C. Longterm antibiotic coverage required
D. Clubbing is usually positive

258. The commonest cause of superior vena caval syndrome is :

A. Sarcoidosis B. Carcinoma lung
C. Retrosternal thyroid D. Coarctation of aorta

259. In respiratory distress syndrome, not seen in :

A. Alveolar pulmonary oxygen ratio less than 0.2
B. X-ray chest shows Bilateral shadows
C. Pulmonary wedge pressure more than 15 mm Hg
D. Lung compliance is decreased

260. Acute respiratory failure with cor pulmonale - findings :

A. Cold entremites B. Headache
C. Small volume pulse D. Bradycardia

261. In an asymptomatic smoker one would find :

A. ↑ closing volume
B. $\uparrow \frac{FEV_1}{FEV}$
C. $\downarrow \frac{FEV_1}{PVC}$
D. ↑ tidal volume

262. The commonest cause of pulmonary embolism :

A. Superficial vein thrombosis

Ans.	254. D	255. D	256. D	257. C	258. B	259. C
	260. E	261. A	262. B			

B. Deep vein thrombosis
C. Pelvic vein thrombosis
D. Heart failure

263. Acute pulmonary oedema and hyperventilation are not seen below the height of :

A. 12,000 feet   B. 15,000 feet
C. 18,000 feet   D. 20,000 feet

264. All of the following is true about pulmonary hypertension except :

A. Soft P2   B. Cyanosis
C. P. pulmonale   D. ↑ Pulmonary artery size

265. The commonest site of lung abscess is :

A. Right upper   B. Right middle
C. Right lower   D. Left lower

266. In a young asthmatic, treatment of choice is injection :

A. Adrenaline   B. Hydrocortisone
C. Promethazine   D. Chlorpheniramine

267. Cholesterol rich pleural effusion is seen in :

A. Nephrotic syndrome   B. Myxoedema
C. SLE   D. Hypercholesterolmia

268. Human body can store oxygen for :

A. 4-10 minutes   B. 15-20 minutes
C. 20-25 minutes   D. 25-30 minutes

269. Wedge pressure in ARDS is usually :

A. Markedly increased   B. Moderately increase
C. Normal   D. Decreased

270. Breath sounds are decreased in following except :

A. Lobar pneumonia   B. Pneumothorax
C. Pleural effusion   D. Atelectasis

271. Least common cause of clubbing is :

A. Adeno ca   B. Sq. cell ca
C. Small cell ca   D. Mesothelioma

272. True about ventillation is :

A. Ventilation perfusion ratio is more at apices
B. ↑ Dead space
C. O2 transport
D. Does not change in Pulmonary embolism

273. Crackling crepitations unaltered by coughing is characteristic of :

A. Pulmonary tuberculosis   B. Interstitial lung disease
C. Klebsiella pneumonia   D. Lung abscess

Ans.	263. A	264. A	265. C	266. A	267. B	268. D
	269. C	270. A	271. C	272. A	273. B	

274. Duchenne's sign is present in :
A. Infantile pneumonia
B. Diaphragmatic palsy
C. Sarcoidosis
D. Muscular dystrophy

275. Hemoptysis is seen :
A. Early in mitral stenosis
B. In VSD
C. Late in mitral stenosis
D. In pulmonary stenosis

276. Pink frothy expectoration is seen in :
A. Pulmonary edema
B. Pulmonary tuberculosis
C. Bronchogenic carcinoma
D. Mucormycosis

277. In Bronchoalveolar lavage, inflammatory cells found in normal individual are ——— X10^6 :
A. Nil
B. 10-30
C. 50-100
D. 100-200

278. Pulmonary hypertension in COPD is due to :
A. Constriction of pulmonary vessels
B. Hypoxia
C. Interstitial fibrosis
D. All of the above

279. Respiratory alkalosis occurs in :
A. Diabetic ketosis
B. Pyloric stenosis
C. Primary aldosteronism
D. Excessive ventilation

280. Pleural aspiration showed ↑ LDH and amylase in :
A. Pulm infarction
B. COPD
C. Pulm. malignancy
D. None of the above

281. Sputum examination from a patient of bronchiectasis is most likely to show :
A. H. influenzae
B. Klebsiella
C. Pseudomonas
D. Anaerobic bacteria

282. Alveolar air in severe pulmonary hypoventilation contains :
A. High PCO2 and high PO2
B. High PCO2 and low PO2
C. Low PCO2 and high PO2
D. Low PCO2 and low PO2

283. Wide alveolar arterial O2 gradient is seen in following except :
A. Bronchiectasis
B. ARDS
C. Interstitial fibrosis
D. Central hypoventilation

Ans. 274. B 275. C 276. A 277. B 278. D 279. D
280. A 281. A 282. C 283. D

284. Sudden onset of cough with increasing dyspnoea in a young adult is due to :

A. Pleural effusion
B. Mycocardial infarction
C. Pulmonary embolism
D. Pneumothorax

285. J receptors are seen in :

A. Aorta
B. Bronchiole
C. Bronchi
D. Alveoli
E. Trachea

286. Type II respiratory failure is seen in :

A. COPD with cor pulmonale
B. Chronic renal failure
C. Adult respiratory distress syndrome
D. Pulmonary fibrosing alveolitis

287. The following are features of Fat Embolism except :

A. Lipemia with purpura
B. Dyspnoea with bilateral pulmonary infiltrate
C. Pulmonary infarction
D. Clouding of consciousness; chorea; joint bends

288. The following statements regarding the one of intravenous Deriphylline in severe asthma are true except :

A. Dose needs modification in presence of congestive Heart failure
B. The drug has wide margin of therapeutic safety
C. Overdose may produce convulsion
D. Arterial oxygen tension may fall after aminophylline administration

289. Emphysema is believed to result from mutation in Alpha-1 antitrypsin gene on chromosome :

A. 12
B. 14
C. 17
D. 19

290. Bovine cough is characteristic of :

A. Acute epiglottitis
B. Tracheitis
C. Laryngeal paralysis
D. Chronic laryngitis
E. Chronic bronchitis

291. The sequence of changes is status asthmaticus is :

I. Respiratory acidosis
II. Respiratory alkalosis
III. Metabolic acidosis
IV. Metabolic alkalosis

A. I, II, III
B. II, I, III
C. I, III, IV
D. II, I, IV

292. Normal intrapleural pressure is :

A. 1 to 2 mm Hg
B. 2 to 4 mm Hg
C. 9.5 to 10 mm Hg
D. -3 to -4 mm Hg

Ans.						
	284. D	**285. D**	**286. A**	**287. C**	**288. B**	**289. B**
	290. C	**291. B**	**292. D**			

293. The physiological dead space is increaed when :

A. Ventilation perfusion ratio is greater than normal
B. Ventilation perfusion ratio is less than normal
C. Hypoxia is present
D. Cyanosis is present

294. A patient of chronic Lt. lung Abscess with generalised Edema, Hypoproteinemia, hepatosplenomegaly without renal failure but reduced urine output. Diagnosis is :

A. Amyloidosis
B. Ch. cor pulmonale with Rt. Heart failure
C. Bronchiectasis
D. Bronchogenic carcinoma

295. Which of the following are the causes of chronic respiratory failure ?

1. Diffuse pulmonary fibrosis
2. Atlantoaxial cervical anomalies
3. Muscular dystrophy
4. Thoaracoplasty

Select the correct answer using the codes given below :
Codes :

A. 1,2 and 3 B. 2,3 and 4
C. 1,3 and 4 D. 1 and 4

296. Which one of the following is not true regarding Klebsiella Pneumonia ?

A. Affect Upper Lobe
B. Produces expansion of lung volume
C. Gentamicin is the antibiotic of choice
D. Does not produce cavitation

297. High oxygen tension in alveoli is due to :

A. Right to left shunt
B. Inappropriate gas exchange
C. Ventilation perfusion mismatch
D. Bronchial asthma

298. Bilateral hilar lymphadenopathy with non caseating granuloma is :

A. Sarcoidosis B. Lymphoma
C. TB D. All of the above

299. Pneumothorax is seen in all except :

A. Eosinophilic granuloma
B. Marfan's syndrome
C. Bronchopulmonary aspergilosis
D. Assisted ventilation

Ans. 293. A 294. A 295. C 296. D 297. C 298. A 299. B

300. True about pulmonary embolism is all except :

A. Most common within two weeks
B. Arises from leg veins
C. Chest pain is commonest symptom
D. More is the survival time, more are chances of recovery

301. In left sided massive pneumothorax, ECG shows following except :

A. Peaked P wave
B. Absent R wave
C. Left axis deviation
D. Precordial T wave inversion

302. In severe bronchial asthma, true is :

A. Infequent rhonchi and absent breath sounds
B. Hyperresonant chest with prolonged expiration
C. Increased fremitus and absent breath sounds
D. Decreased fremitus and crackles

303. All of the following are features of sarcoidosis except :

A. Joint involvement
B. Hepatosplenomegaly
C. Low levels of serum complement
D. Erythema nodosum

304. Adult Respiratory Distress Syndrome (ARDS) is diagnosed by all of the following characteristics except :

A. Dyspnoea and tachypnoea in a patient of trauma, shock or sepsis
B. Arterial hypoxemia
C. Hypercapnia
D. Diffuse alveolar and interstitial infiltrates on X-ray chest

305. The Reid Index (ratio of the thickness of submucosal glands to that of bronchial wall) is characteristically increased in :

A. Bronchiectasis
B. Bronchogenic carcinoma
C. Chronic bronchial asthma
D. Chronic bronchitis

306. Bronchial asthma may be complicated by infection with :

A. Aspergillus fumigatus
B. Mucormycosis
C. Micropolyspora faeni
D. Candida albicans

307. True about obstructive lung disease is all except :

A. ↓ vital capacity
B. ↑ residual capacity
C. ↑ FEV1/FVC
D. ↓ Tidal volume

308. Severity of bronchial asthma is indicated by :

A. RR-24/min
B. Pulse - 110/min
C. Pulsus paradoxus 15 mm Hg
D. FEV1/FVC is 75%

Ans.						
	300. C	301. B	302. B	303. C	304. C	305. D
	306. A	307. C	308. C			

309. Tropical pulmonary eosinophilia is characterized by all except :

A. Eosinophilia 3000/mm3

B. Prominent Wheeze

C. Bilateral mottling in chest X-ray

D. Hypersensitivity to ascariasis

310. Arterial blood gas data in a young girl on admission shows the following changes :

PO_2 104 mm Hg.

O_2 saturation 99%

PCO_2 24 mm Hg.

HCO_3 12 mmHg and

pH = 7.25

The most likely diagnosis is :

A. Acute severe bronchial asthma

B. Diabetic ketoacidosis

C. Hysterical hyperventilation

D. Ethanol ingestion

311. The following are features of hypersensitivity pneu-monitis, except :

A. Neutrophils

B. Eosinophilia

C. Lymphopenia

D. ESR

312. Bronchial breath sounds and Aegophony in a patient with pericardial effusion is known as :

A. Levine's sign

B. Kussamaul's sign

C. Ewart's sign

D. Hill's sign

313. In the management of acute severe asthma all of the following statement are true except :

A. Beta-2 agonist aerosol therapy is very useful

B. Costicosteroids are useful in preventing relapse

C. Acidosis decreases the responsiveness to bronchodilators

D. Disodium Chromoglycate is helpful in remitting the attack

314. The management of spontaneous pneumothorax only slight retraction of the lung and minimal symptoms, should be :

A. Single needle aspiration

B. Thoracic pump

C. Multiple needle aspiration

D. Observation

Ans. **309. B** **310. C** **311. B** **312. C** **313. D** **314. D**

315. Fever, Tachycardia. Respiratory distress and a non-productive cough occuring within 48 hours after abdominal operation in an obese male would most likely be due to :

A. Pneumonia B. Pulmonary infarction

C. Myocardial infarction D. Atelectasis

316. Diagnostic features of bronchopulmonary aspergillosis may include :

1. Peripheral blood eosinophilia
2. Elevated IgE levels
3. Central bronchiectasis
4. History of brownish plug in the sputum.

Select the correct answer using the codes given below :

Codes :

A. 1, 2, 3 and 4 B. 1, 3 and 4

C. 2 and 3 D. 1, 2 and 4

317. Consider the following statements regarding pneumonia :

1. The roentgenographic features of non-segmental consolidation with air bronchogram is a feature of pneumococcal pneumonia
2. In pneumococcal pneumonia, sputum on gram staining may show grain-positive lancet shaped diplococci
3. *Pneumocystis carinii* pneumonia is common in AIDS patients
4. There may be hypoxemia, hypocarbia and respiratory alkalosis.

Which of these statements are correct ?

A. 1, 2, 3 and 4 B. 2, 3 and 4

C. 1, 2 and 3 D. 1 and 4

318. Consider the following statements regarding pneumonia :

1. Pneumococcal pneumonia is characterised by homogeneous consolidation of one or more lobes of the lungs.
2. Legionella pneumonia is caused by a bacillus
3. Primary viral pneumonia is most frequently due to influenza virus
4. Pneumonia due to opportunistic infections is seen in immunocompromised host

Which of the above statements are correct ?

A. 1 and 4 B. 1 and 2

C. 2,3 and 4 D. 1,2,3 and 4

W319. Not a feature of acute severe asthma :

A. Tachycardia B. Respiratory alkalosis

C. Pulsus paradoxus D. Cyanosis

Ans.	315. D	316. B	317. A	318. D	319. NONE
	320. B				

320. 35 year old man with cadavaric renal presents allograft on azathioprine presents with fever, cough sputum shows, long crook branching beaded gram positive filaments, treatment is

A. Cefalexin
B. Erythromycin
C. Sulphosaxazole
D. Cotrimoxazole

321. Treatment of Pulmonary edema is all except :

A. IV fluids
B. Furosemide IV
C. Morphine
D. O2

322. A female patient with high fever, vomiting, diarrhea confusion, and increased bilirubin, hyponatremia and lower lobe infiltrates cause is :

A. Streptococcus pneumoniae
B. Legionella
C. Staph aureus
D. Pseudonomas

323. Match List I (Lesion) with List II (Precipitating factor) and select the correct answer using the codes given below the Lists :

List I	List II
a. Cavitatory lung lesion	1. Acute pancreatitis
b. Eosinophilic pneumonia	2. Staphylococcal pneumonias
c. Hilar lymphadenopathy	3. Nitrofurantoin therapy
d. Adult respiratory distress syndrome	4. Sarcoidosis

Codes :

	a	b	c	d
A.	2	1	4	3
B.	2	3	4	1
C.	3	1	2	4
D.	4	3	2	1

324. An adult patient of pulmonary tuberculosis, on drug treatment, complains of diminution of vision. The drug causing this condition is:

A. Isoniazid
B. Rifampicin
C. Ethambutol
D. Pyrazinamide

325. The maximum period required for postexposure chemoprophylaxis for HIV is:

A. 4 Weeks
B. 6 Weeks
C. 8 Weeks
D. 12 Weeks

Ans. **321. A** **322. B** **323. B** **324. C** **325. D**

326. Transudative pleural effusion is caused by :

A. VA Sclerotherapy B. Bypass surgery
C. Radiation therapy D. Peritoneal dialysis

327. A 55-year old male chronic smoker complains of cough, mild haemoptysis and weight loss of 5 kg in 3 months. Physical examination reveals clubbing of fingers and signs of collapse of right lower lobe. Chest X-ray reveals mass in hilum of right lung. The most likely diagnosis is :

A. Pulmonary tuberculosis B. Bronchogenic carcinoma
C. Pneumococcal pneumonia D. Sarcoidosis

328. Blurring of right border occurs in which broncho-pulmonary segment atlectasis :

A. Right upper lobe apical segment
B. Right upper lobe anterior segment
C. Right middle lobe
D. Right lower lobe

329. Which of the statements is not true regarding Macleod's Syndrome ?

A. It is not a true emphysema
B. Occurs before 8 years of age
C. It is unilateral emphysema
D. The pulmonary artery on the affected side is hyperplastic
E. It is also called Swyer-Jame's Syndrome

330. Amylase increased in pleural fluid is seen in following except :

A. Rheumatoid arthritis B. Esophageal perforation
C. Malignancy D. Gall stone pancreatitis

331. All following secreted by bronchogenic Ca A/E :

A. Nor adrenaline B. 5 HT
C. ACTH D. ADH

332. Asbestos maximally produces :

A. Mesothelioma B. Bronchogenic carcinoma
C. Bronchial adenoma D. Sarcoma

333. A worker working in cotton industry presents with night cramps, sweating & cough. Likely cause is :

A. Interstital lung disease B. Rest after 5 days of work
C. Pulm. edema D. COPD

334. Choice of drug by inhalation in acute asthma not responding to salbutamol is :

A. Ipratropium bromide B. Atropine sulfate
C. Isopropamide D. Hyoscine methyl bromide

Ans.	326. D	327. B	328. B	329. D	330. A	331. A
	332. A	333. D	334. A			

335. A patient comes with sudden repiratory distress, on examination bilateral basal crepts are present over chest suggestive of pulmonary edema with normal alveolar wedge pressure. The likely cause is :

A. Myocardial Infarction B. Congestive heart failure
C. Narcotic overdose D. Cardiogenic shock

336. A patient comes with nonproductive cough, hemoptysis and grade III clubbing chest X-ray shows upper left zone lesion. The likely cause is :

A. Small cell carcinoma lung
B. Tuberculosis
C. Non-small cell carcinoma lung
D. Fungal infection of lung

337. A patient develops acute respiratory distress, stridor, hyperinflation on one side of chest with decreased breath sound on that side. Most likely cause is :

A. Foreign body aspiration B. Aspiration pneumonia
C. Asthma D. Pleural effusion

338. Blood gas measurements of a patient shows the following valures pH 7.2 p CO2 80 mm Hg, pO2 46 mmHg. Which of the following could be the most probable diagnosis :

A. Acute asthma B. Acute exacerbation of COPD
C. ARDS D. Severe pneumonia

339. A man presents with non productive cough for 4weeks, grade III class and apical lobe lesion onX-ray. Diagnosis ?

A. Small cell carcinoma B. Non small cell carcinoma
C. Fungal infection D. Tuberculosis

340. Pulm edema associated with normal PCWP. Which of the followings is cause :

A. High altitude
B. Narcotics overdose
C. Post cardiopulm bypass
D. Bilateral renal artery stenosis

341. All of the following are true about type I respiratory f ailure except :

A. Decreased PaO2 B. Decreased PaCO2
C. Normal PaCO2 D. Normal P(A-a) O2 gradient

342. A man presents with fever, weight loss and cough. Mantoux is 17 x 19 mm and sputum cytology negative for AFB. Diagnosis is :

A. Pulmonary TB B. Fungal infection
C. Viral pneumonia D. Mycoplasma pneumonia

Ans.	335. C	336. C	337. A	338. B	339. B	340. D
	341. D	342. A				

W343. A diabetic female on INH and rifampin for TB suffers DVT; started warfarin; PT is not raised; next step :

A. Long term heparin therapy
B. Increase dose of warfarin
C. Switch ethambutol for rifampin
D. Use LMW heparin

344. **Exudative pleural effusion is not seen in :**

A. Cirrhosis liver B. Pulmonary embolism
C. Nephrotic syndrome D. Peritoneal dialysis

345. All the following are poor prognostic factors in community acquired pneumonia except :

A. Temp > 102 F B. Resp. rate > 30
C. Diastolic BP < 60 mmHg D. BUN > 20 mg

346. In treatment of ARDS O2 conc kept at which level ? :

A. 20-40 mmHg B. 40-60 mmHg
C. 50-100 D. 60-80

347. Pan acinar emphysema occur in all except :

A. Smoking B. α-1 antitrypsim deficiency
C. Both D. None

348. In hemoptysis all are true except :

A. >100 ml 24 hrs is severe
B. Rigid bronchoscopy for diagnosis
C. Unaffected lower lung region
D. Treatment with antibiotics

349. A patient presented with hemoptysis and persistent cough. The chest X-ray of the patient was normal. the next best investigation is :

A. Helical CT B. High resolution CT
C. Bronchoscopy D. Angiography

350. A patient had acute pulmonary embolism. Echocardiography showed right ventricular hypokinesia with tricuspid regurgitation. The treatment to l given is :

A. LMWH B. Thrombolytic therapy
C. IVC filters D. Anticoagulants

351. A patient presented with cough. The mantoux was 19 x 17 mm. Sputum examination was negative for acid-fast bacilli. The diagnosis is most likely to be :

A. Pulmonary tuberculosis B. Pneumococcal pneumonia
C. Mycoplasma pneumonia D. Viral pneumonia

Ans.	343. C,D	344. B	345. D	346. B	347. B	348. D
	349. B	350. B	351. A			

352. **'Calcification of diaphragmatic pleura' is characteristic of pneumoconioses due to:**
A. Asbestosis
B. Berylliosis
C. Silicosis
D. Anthracosis

353. **Honey comb lung is seen all except :**
A. Tuberous sclerosis
B. Rheumatoid arthritis
C. Histiocytosis
D. Wegener's granulomatosis

354. **Statement true about mycoplasma penumonia is :**
A. Most commonly seen in 2-5 years age group
B. Frequently leads to lung abscess
C. Symptoms are severe but signs in the chest are scanty
D. None of the above

355. **Air way obstruction in emphysema is due to :**
A. Mucosal edema
B. Submucosal muscularis hypertrophy
C. Loss of elastic recoil of lung
D. Mucosal hyperplasia

356. **The following is an example of type I respiratory failure ?**
A. Narcotic overdose
B. ARDS
C. Primary alveolar hypoventilation
D. Chronic bronchitis

357. **All the following are causes of hemorrhagic pleural effusion except :**
A. Pulmonary embolism
B. Rheumatoid arthritis
C. Pancreatitis
D. TB

358. **Hypersensitivity pneumonitis is seen in :**
A. Bagassosis
B. Sarcoidosis
C. Berrylliosis
D. Silicosis

359. **While inserting a central venous catheter, a pateint develops respiratory distress. The most likely cause is :**
A. Hemothorax
B. Penumothorax
C. Pleural effusion
D. Hypovolumia

360. **A patient has presented to you with pleural effusion. The best site of aspiration of the fluid would be through the :**
A. 5th intercostal space in the midclavicular line
B. 2th intercostal space close to the sternum
C. 7th intercostal space in mid axillary line
D. 10th intercostal space in paravertebral location

Ans.	352. A	353. D	354. C	355. C	356. B	355. B
	358. A	359. B	360. C			

361. Asthma is differentiated from obstructive lung disease with emphysema in the laboratory by the demonstration of :

A. Normal spirometry
B. Positive skin allergy tests to pollens
C. Broncho provocation test with methacholine
D. Normal diffusion capacity in the presence of airway obstruction

362. Which of the following abnormality in lung function is not found in emphysema :

A. Decreased vital capacity B. Increased residual volume
C. Decreased PEFR D. Increased FEV1

363. In a person exposed to the asbestos, which of the following lesion is visible earliest in relation to time interval between exposure and development of lesion :

A. Pleural mesothelioma B. Pleural effusion
C. Pleural plaque D. Bronchial carcinoma

364. A 30 year-old male patient rapidly rises to an altitude of 18,000 feet and he does not develop breath lessness. All of the following changes occur except :

A. Decreased barometric pressure
B. Increased O2 release from hemoglobin
C. Increased diffusion capacity
D. Increased erythropoietin secretion

365. Immediate phase of the bronchial asthma is mediated by the :

A. Macrophages B. Lymphocytes
C. Mast cells D. Neutrophils

366. Pulmonary edema with cardiomegaly is seen in :

A. Mitral stenosis B. Mitral regurgitation
C. Aortic stenosis D Hypertrophic cardiomyopathy

367. All of the following conditions may predispose to Pulmonary embolism except :

A. Protein S deficiency B. Malignancy
C. Obesity D. Progesterone therapy

368. A patient while undergoing scalene node biopsy suddenly developed cyanosis, breathlessness, tachypnea & tachycardia with absent breath sound on the side of biopsy. What is the best next treatment ?

A. Endracheal intubation B. Oxygen support
C. I.P.P.V. D. Intercostal drain

369. Following cranial nerve is most commonly involved in patients with sarcoidosis :

A. II Cranial nerve B. III Cranial nerve
C. VII Cranial nerve D. IX Cranial nerve

Ans.	361. D	362. D	363. C	364. C	365. C	366. B
	367. D	368. D	369. C			

370. In type-II respiratory failure, there is :

A. Low pO2 and low pCO2

B. Low pO2 and high pCO2

C. Normal pO2 and high pCO2

D. Low pO2 and normal pCO2

371. The most common cause of acute corpulmonale is :

A. Pneumonia

B. Pulmonary thrombo-embolism

C. Chronic obstructive pulmonary disease

D. Primary spontaneous pneumothorax

372. All the following diseases are associated with peripheral blood eosinophilia except :

A. Allergic bronchopulmonary aspergillosis (ABPA)

B. Loffler's syndrome

C. Pulmonary eosinophilic granuloma

D. Churg-Strauss syndrom

373. Hemoptysis may occur in all of the following conditious except :

A. Pulmonary embolism B. Pulmonary tuberculosis

C. Pulmonary stenosis D. Mitral stenosis

374. Consider the following statements :

The features of severe asthma include

1. Central cyanosis
2. Disturbance of consciousness
3. Pulsus paradoxus
4. Heart rate less than 60/minute

Which of these statemnts are correct :

A. 2, 3 and 4 B. 1, 3 and 4

C. 1,2 and 3 D. 1, 2 and 4

375. A patient presents with breathlessness. He has bilateral basal crepitations. Lung function tests reveal decrease in total lung capacity (TLC) and vital capacity (VC) with normal FEV/VC ratio. The most likely diagnosis is :

A. Chronic bronchitis

B. Idiopathic pulmonary fibrosis

C. Cystic fibrosis

D. Allergic bronchopulmonary aspergillosis

Ans.	370. B	371. B	372. C	373. C	374. C	375. B

376. Match List I (Respiratory sign) with List II (Clinical condition) and select the correct answer using the codes given below the Lists :

List I (Respiratory sign)	List II (Clinical condition)
a. Localized wheeze	1. Pleural effusion
b. Shifting dullness	2. Empyema
c. Ellis curve	3. Hydropneumothorax
d. Intercostal tenderness	4. Bronchial tumour

Codes :

	A	B	C	D
A.	2	1	3	4
B.	4	3	1	2
C.	2	3	1	4
D.	4	1	3	2

377. The blood gas parameters pH 7.58, pCO2 23 mm Hg, pO2 300 mmHg and oxygen saturation 60% are most consistent with :

A. Carbonmonoxide poisoning
B. Ventilatory malfunction
C. Voluntary hyperventilation
D. Methyl alcohol poisoning

378. The diffusion capacity of Lung (DLco) is decreased in all of the following conditions except :

A. Interstitial lung disease B. Good pasture's syndrome
C. Emphysema D. Primary pulmonary hypertension

379. A 62 years old man with caracioma of lung presented to emergency department with respiratory distress. His EKG showed electrical alternans. The most likely diagnosis is :

A. Pneumothorax. B. Pleural effusion.
C. Cardiac tamponade. D. Constrictive pericarditis.

380. A middle aged old man, with chronic renal failure is diagnosed to have sputum positive pulmonary tuberculosis. His creatinine clearance is 25ml/min. All of the following drugs need modification in doses except :

A. Isoniazid B. Streptomycin
C. Rifampicin D. Ethambutol.

Ans. **376. B** **377. A** **378. B** **379. C** **380. C**

381. An obese lady aged 45 years, was brought to emergency in a semi comatose condition. The laboratory investigations showed K+ (5.8 mmol/L); Na+ (136 mmol/L); blood pH (7.1), HCO3 (12 mmol/L),' ketone bodies (350 mg/dl). The expected level of blood glucose for this lady is:

A. < 45 mg/dl.
B. < 120 mg/dl.
C. >180 mg/dl.
D. < 75 mg/dl.

382. A 9- years old boy has steroid dependent nephrotic syndrome for the last 5 years. He has received corticosteroids almost continuously during this period and has cushingoid features. The blood pressure is 120/86 mmHg and there are bilateral subcapsular cataracts. The treatment of choice is:

A. Levamisole.
B. Cyclophosphamide.
C. Cyclosporin A.
D. Intravenous pulse corticosteroids.

383. A woman is admitted with complaints of low-grade fever of 6 weeks duration. Chest radiograph reveals bihilar adenopathy with clear lung fields. All of the following investigations will be useful in differential diagnosis except?

A. CD4/CD8 counts in the blood
B. Serum ACE levels
C. CECT of chest
D. Gallium scan

384. The level of which one of the followign compounds is elevated in bronchial asthma ?

A. PGI2
B. PGH2
C. Leukotriens
D. Thromboxane

385. Which one of the following organs should always be imaged in a suspected case of bronchogenic carcinoma :

A. Adrenals
B. Kidneys
C. Spleen
D. Pancreas

386. Serum angiotensin converting enzyme may be raised in all of the following except :

A. Sarcoidosis
B. Silicosis
C. Berylliosis
D. Bronchogenic carcinoma

387. The abnormal preoperative pulmonary function test in a patient with severe kyphoscoliosis includes :

A. Increased RV/TLC
B. Reduced FEV/FAC
C. Reduced FEV
D. Increased FRC

Ans.	381. C	382. B	383. A	384. C	385. A	386. D
	387. A					

388. Iprotropium bromide is useful in bronchial asthma because of :
A. Anticholinergic effect
B. Vasodilator properties
C. Antiallergic action
D. Stabilization of mast cells

389. Mainstay of treatment in acute severe bronchial asthma is :
A. Local acting steroids
B. Local acting β_1 agonist
C. Theophylline
D. Oral steroids

390. Drug which interferes with metabolism of theophylline is :
A. EM
B. Gentamicin
C. Penicillin
D. Furazolidine

391. Of the following which is useful in acute asthma :
A. Cromolyn
B. Corticosteroids
C. Ketotifen
D. Terbutaline

392. Which of the following drug is not useful in treatment of acute attack of bronchial asthma :
A. Nifedipine
B. Orciprenaine
C. Salbutamol
D. Theophylline

393. Steroid given by inhalation is :
A. Dexamethasone
B. Hydrocortisone
C. Triamcilone
D. Beclamethason

394. All of the following except one suppresses cough :
A. Acetylcysteine
B. Benzonatate
C. Codeine
D. Chlorcyclizine

395. If one cannot differentiate between cardiac and respiratory asthma, the drug to be avoided is :
A. Steroid
B. Antibiotic
C. Morphine
D. Beta blocker

396. Rapid infusion of intravenous aminophylline may cause :
A. Tachycardia
B. Hypotension
C. Convulsions
D. Hypertension

397. In chronic obstructive airway disease following are used except :
A. Bromhexine
B. Deriphylline
C. Steam inhalation
D. 100% O2

398. Aminophylline acts by :
A. Stabilizing membrane of mast cells
B. Decreasing phosphodiesterase activity
C. Directly on smooth muscle
D. By releasing catecholeamines

399. Which of the following is not an expectorant :
A. Codeine
B. Bicarbonates
C. Iodide
D. Ipecacuanua

Ans.	388.A	389. B	390. A	391. D	392. A	393. D
	394. A	395. D	396. A	397. D	398. B	399. A

400. Local anesthetic antitussive :
A. Noscapine B. Dextromethorphan
C. Carbetapentane D. Benzonatate

401. The drug used in bronchial asthma is :
A. Cimetidine B. Methyl xanthine
C. Propranolol D. Dihydroxy quinoline

402. Regarding aminophylline infusion, incorrect is :
A. Contractility of diaphragm
B. O2 tension in blod
C. Low dose required in smokers
D. Inter action with concurrent erythromycin therapy

403. True for sodium cromoglycate is :
A. Used in acute bronchial asthma
B. Stabilized the mast cells
C. Inhibits one action of chemical mediators
D. Inhibits the chemotaxis

404. Beta blockers used in bronchial asthma exert action by :
A. Selective β1 agonism B. Selective β2 agonism
C. Selective β1 antagonism D. Selective β2 antagonism

405. Bronchodilator effect without significant cardiac stimulation is the characteristic of :
A. Isoprenaline B. Isoxuprine
C. Propranolol D. Salbutamol

406. Corticosteroids are useful in status asthmaticus primarly because :
A. They are potent directly acting bronchodilator
B. They mimic dilator neurotransmitters
C. They antagonise the released mediators
D. They bring about a non-specific reduction in inflammatory response

407. Thecphyline causes following except :
A. Bronchodilatation B. Gastric irritation
C. Depresses C.N.S. D. Potentiates sympathomimetics

408. Theophylline overdosage may produce all of the following except :
A. Acute renal failure B. Rhabdomyolysis
C. Rise in SGPT D. Hypotension

409. Longest acting bronchodilator is :
A. Salbutamol B. Bitolterol
C. Rimiteral D. Ritodrine

410. Drug of choice in Theophylline poisoning :
A. Cortisone B. Propranolol
C. Thyroxine D. Phenobarbitone

Ans.	400. D	401. B	402. C	403. B	404. B	405. B
	406. B	407. C	408. A	409. B	410. B	

411. Aerosolized ribavirin is used in the treatment of brondchiolitis :
A. RSV
B. H. influenza
C. Pneumococcus
D. Streptococcus

412. Antitussives act by :
A. Liuefying bronchial secretions
B. Raising the threshold of courgh centre
C. Reducing cough inducing impusles from the lungs
D. Both (B) and (C)

413. The common and dose related side effect of Salbutamol is :
A. Rise in blood pressure
B. Muscle tremor
C. Hyperglycaemia
D. Central nervous system stimulation

414. An asthmatic patient is on theophylline suddenly developed infection, which of the following antibiotic should not be given to prevent side effects of theo- phylline :
A. Erythromycin
B. Ampicillin
C. Cephalexin
D. Sparfloxacin

415. All are true regarding treatment with aminophylline except :
A. It decreases the oxygen tension
B. Its dose is to be decreased in smokers
C. It increases the contractility of the diaphragm
D. Interaction with erythromycin can increase its toxicity

416. Correct about theophylline is :
A. t1/2 is less in CHF
B. t1/2 is less in smoker
C. t1/2 is less in obst. jaundice
D. t1/2 is less in bronchila asthma

417. A patient taking Theophyline develops chest infection. Which of the following drugs would increase the toxicity of Theophylline :
A. Sparfloxacin
B. Erythromycin
C. Cephalexin
D. Amoxicillin

418. Name an electrolyte disturbance that may follow nebulization with salbutamol :
A. Hyponatrimia
B. Hypernatrimia
C. Hypokalemia
D. Hypocalcemia

419. Child with bronchial asthma, steroid should be given as :
A. Subcutaneous
B. Aerosol
C. Intravenous
D. Oral

Ans.	411. A	412. D	413. B	414. A	415. B	416. A
	417. B	418. C	419. B			

420. A neonate delivered at 32 weeks, on ventilator, xray shows white shadow and reveals SpO2 of 75, ventilator settings are as, Fi O2 70, rate 50/minute step to be taken ?

A. Increase rate to 60
B. Increase rate to 60
C. Continue with the same
D. Weaning ventilator

421. A neonate presents with respiratory distress, contralateral mediastinal and multiple cystic air filled lesions in chest. Most likely diagnosis is :

A. Congenital diaphragmatic hernia
B. Congenital lung cysts
C. Pneumonia
D. Hyaline membrane disease

422. Surfactant production in lungs starts at :

A. 28 weeks
B. 32 wks
C. 34 wks
D. 36 wks

423. 3 month old child presents with intermittent stridor. Most likely cause is :

A. Laryngotracheobronchitis
B. Laryngomalacia
C. Foreign body in larynx
D. Laryngeal papilloma

424. The following are features of transient tachypnea of newborn, except :

A. Seen in early neonatal period
B. May be associated with grunting & cyanosis
C. May be associated with crepts & wheez
D. Interlobar effusion is present

425. Transient tachypnoea of new born is seen in :

A. Forceps delivery
B. Elective caesarean section
C. Ventouse extraction
D. Normal vaginal delivery

426. In a newborn with respiratory distress syndrome, all the following are true except :

A. Increased incidence in <34 weeks
B. More common in infants of diabetic mothers
C. 100% oxygen is given in treatment
D. Cyanosis is present

427. Trendelenberg test is for testing which action at hip :

A. Flexion
B. Extention
C. Abduction
D. Adduction

Ans.	420. D	421. B	422. A	423. B	424. B	425. B
	426. C	427. C				

428. Rattling sound in a child is produced due to :

A. Obstruction in oropharynx
B. Obstruction in trachea & larynx
C. Obstruction in bronchi & bronchioles
D. Secretions in bronchi & bronchioles

429. A 5-year old boy, a known patient of bronchial asthma, presents with cough, wheezing and breathlessness. Examination shows respiratory rate 48/minute, pulsus oparadoxus and bilateral rhonchi. The most appropriate immediate treatment is :

A. Intravenous theophylline and corticosteroids
B. Intravenous theophylline and nubulized salbutamol
C. Nebulized salbutamol and ipratropinm
D. Nebulized salbutamol and intraenous corticosteroids

430. Consider the following statements :
Breath holding spells in children have the following feature.

1. They are preceded by minor trauma
2. Child stops breathing and is cyanosed
3. Child becomes suddenly pale and limp
4. Frequency becomes less on zinc supplementation

Which of the above statements are correct :

A. 1, 2 and 3
B. 1 and 2
C. 2, 3 and 4
D. 1, 3 and 4

431. A child aged 24 months was brought to the Primary health centre with complaints of cough and fever for the past 2 days. On examination, the child weighed 11 kg, respiratory rate was 38/min chest indrawing was present. The most appropriate management for this patient is :

A. Classify as pneumonia and refer urgently to secondary level hospital
B. Classify as pneumonia, start antibiotics and advise to report after 2 days
C. Classify as severe pneumonia, start antibiotics and refer urgently
D. Classify as severe pneumonia and refer urgently

432. In a 7 years child, trachea would be shifted away from affected side in all, except :

A. Massive atelectasis
B. Tension pneumothorax
C. Tension pleural effusion
D. Masive emphysema

433. In a child with exercise induced asthma, true is :

A. Prophylaxis with steroids
B. Prophylaxis with β_1 agonists
C. Prophylaxis with theophyline
D. Breathing exercises

Ans.	428. D	429. D	430. A	431. C	432. A	433. B

434. Child with which of the following throat infection needs systemic antibiotic therapy :

A. Pneumococci
B. β haemolytic streptococci
C. Staph. aureus
D. All of the above

435. Usual feature of Pneumonia in a child is :

A. Cyanosis
B. Resp rate 60/mt
C. Temp 103°F
D. Gastric dilatation

436. Primary site of T.B. in a child :

A. Ghon focus
B. Intestinal
C. Skin
D. Miliary

437. Surfactant type II deficiency leads to :

A. Hyaline Membrane Disease
B. Fine mottling
C. B/L crepts changing with coughing
D. None

438. A child with bronchiolitis - about treatment not true is :

A. Humidified oxygen
B. Anti pyretics if fever
C. Antibiotics if child is toxic and B/L rales
D. Antibiotics not required

439. Dyspnea with unilateral translucency of Hemithorax in a 1 day old infant is suggestive of :

A. Pneumatocele
B. Diaphragmatic hernia
C. Multiple cogenital cysts
D. Cystic fibrosis

440. Characteristic features of pneumococcal pneumoniae include all except :

A. Meningism
B. Delrium
C. Petechial rash
D. Hypochondrial pain

441. Characteristics of tuberculous pleural effusion include each of the following, except :

A. Rare before the age of 5 years
B. Supposed to result from discharge of caseous material of a peripheral primary focus or enlarged regional lymph node
C. Symptoms include fever, weightloss, chest pain an dyspnea
D. Vocal fremitus is increased

442. Characteristics of miliary tuberculosis include each of the following, except :

A. Onset is usually insidious
B. Chest signs may be absolutely absent
C. X-ray chest has snow-storm appearance
D. Toxemia is frequently marked

Ans.	434. D	435. B	436. A	437. A	438. B	439. A
	440. C	441. D	442. D			

443. The commonest cause of haemoptysis in childhood is :

A. Mitral stenosis B. Bronchiectasis
C. Pertussis D. Tuberculosis

444. In miliary tuberculosis, the method of spread is :

A. Lymphatic B. Intra bronchial
C. Contiguous D. Haematogenous

445. Which of the following conditions is least likely to be responsible for neonatal stridor :

A. Congenital goitre B. Cretinism
C. Birth trauma D. Pierre-Robin syndrome

446. The most important drug in the treatment of primary pulmonary tuberculosis in children is :

A. Rifampicin B. Isoniazide
C. Streptomycin D. PAS

447. A newborn has signs of respiratory distress. X-ray reveals : generalised haziness of both lungs, superimposed noduloreticular pattern of increased density, the lumens of largest bronchi stand out as conspicuous air shadows. The most probable diagnosis is :

A. Hyaline membrane disease
B. Intrauterine pneumonia
C. Massive emphysema
D. Massive atelectasis

448. Which of the following is an indication for tonsillectomy ?

A. Asthma
B. Rheumatic fever
C. Glomerulonephritis
D. Persistent carrier of diphtheria bacilli

449. Pleurisy in primary tuberculosis is :

A. Never observed B. Very common
C. Extremely rare D. Seen only among adults

450. Chronic and recurrent pneumonia are common in all of the following, except :

A. Hyperglobulinaemia B. Agammaglobulinaemia
C. Cystic fibrosis of pancrea D. Rheumatic fever

451. Pulmonary haemosiderosis is a feature of :

A. Goodpasture's syndrome
B. Thrombocytopenic prupura
C. Myocarditis, cow's milk hypersensitivity
D. All are true

Ans.	443. B	444. D	445. B	446. B	447. A	448. D
	449. B	450. D	451. D			

452. **What is the long term recognised complication of O2 therapy in newborn ?**

A. Atelectasis and retrolental fibroplasia
B. Cerebral palsy
C. Bronchiectasis
D. High tone deafness

453. **Croup syndrome is usually caused by :**

A. Rhinoviruses B. Coxsackie A virus
C. Coxsackie B virus D. Para influenza viruses

454. **A persistent, bloody, purulent nasal discharge suggests :**

A. Syphilis B. Measles
C. Poliomyelitis D. Allergic rhinitis

455. **Streptococcal pharyngitis is most frequently associated with :**

A. Hoarseness B. Cough
C. Rhinitis D. Diffuse redness of tonsils

456. **In staphylococcal pneumonia, acute respiratory distress is due to:**

A. Pneumatocele formation B. Tension pneumothorax
C. Pleural effusion D. Spreading pneumonia

457. **Respiratory syncitial virus causes all except :**

A. Cold in children B. Coryza in adults
C. Pneumonia in elderly D. Acute Resp. distress syndrome

458. **Which of the following is true of bronchiolitis except :**

A. Caused by RSV B. Occurs in school age
C. Leads to asthma D. Treatment is oxygen

459. **A newborn infant is observed to be cyanotic and tachypnoeic. He is placed in 100% O2 and the cyanosis clears completely. The infant most likely has :**

A. CNS disease
B. Liver disease
C. Cyanotic congenital heart disease
D. Lung disease

460. **Respiratory distress syndrome type II has the following features except :**

A. Hypoxia & Hypocapnia
B. Tachypnoea and Cyanosis
C. Lungs show rales and rhonchi
D. Recover within 3-4 hours

Ans. 452. A 453. D 454. A 455. D 456. B 457. D
458. B 459. D 460. D

461. What is true of 'Canals of Lambert' in the alveolar spaces of the lung :

A. Bronchio Alveolar connections
B. Prevent atelectasis
C. Delay in collapse
D. All of the above

462. A newborn infant coughs and gets cyanosed soon after ingesting fluids. There is no difficulty in swallowing, coarse rhonchi and rales are there after swallowing. There is gastric distension after crying but no symptoms after lavage feedings. The most likely diagnosis is :

A. Achalasia
B. Pyloric stenosis
C. Isolated oesophageal atresia
D. Tracheoesophageal fistula without oesophageal atresia

463. Most important factor predisposing to respiratory distress syndrome (RDS) :

A. Cold stress
B. Prematurity
C. Hypoglycemia
D. Precipitous delivery

464. Untreated infants with severe R D S usually develop :

A. Metabolic acidosis
B. Respiratory alkalosis
C. Respiratory acidosis and metabolic acidosis
D. Respiratory alkalosis and metabolic alkalosis

465. The lecithin-sphinogomyelin ratio of amniotic fluid is a useful indicator of the maturity of foetal :

A. Liver
B. Kidney
C. Lungs
D. C N S

466. A lecithin-sphingomyelin ratio (greater than 2) generally indicates that the foetus :

A. Does not have intrauterine pneumonia
B. Will be able to breath spontaenously at birth
C. Will nto develop idiopathic respiratory distress syndrome
D. None of the above

467. The major site of right to left shunting in respiratory distress syndrome is :

A. In liver
B. In lungs
C. At ductus arteriosus
D. At foramen ovale

468. Most important agent in therapy of R D S is :

A. Lecithin
B. Ampicillin
C. Digitalis
D. Oxygen

Ans. 461. D 462. D 463. B 464. C 465. C 466. C 467. B 468. D

469. Following are early signs of RDS in a child except :

A. RR more than 6 of min
B. Cyanosed at ram temperature
C. Sternal regression and droping in
D. Signs of shock grunting respiration

470. Each of the following pneumonia occurs in the basal portion of lungs (lower lobes), except for :

A. Klebsiella pneumonia
B. Mycoplasma pneumonia
C. Pneumococcal pneuomonia
D. Viral pneumonia

471. Which of the following organisms is most commonly associated with AIDS pneumonia ?

A. Klebsiella
B. Streptococcus pneumoniae
C. Mycoplasma pneumoniae
D. Mycobactecium tuberculosis

472. Pneumatocele is commonly found in cases of :

A. Pneumococcal pneumonia
B. Streptococcal pneumonia
C. Klebsiella pneumonia
D. H. influezae pneumonia
E. None of the above

473. The major advantage of alternate day prednisone therapy for conditions such as asthma is :

A. There is less adrenal suppression
B. More effective
C. More convenient
D. Less expensive

474. All ar true regarding Staphylococcal pneumonia, except :

A. Uncommon below the age of 5 years
B. Pneumatoceles are pathognomonic
C. Abdomen is usually distended with ileus
D. Evidence of infection elsewhere in the body

475. What is the most efficient way to confirm pneumothorax :

A. Chest X-ray
B. Chest tube insertion
C. Measuring tidal volumes
D. Aspiration in Anterior axillary line

476. Which of the following is not true about bronchiectasis :

A. Increased incidence in rheumatoid arthritis
B. Streptococcus is the most common organism causing infection
C. Longterm antibiotic coverage required
D. Clubbing is usually positive

Ans.	469. C	470. A	471. D	472. C	473. A	474. A
	475. D	476. C				

477. The commonest symptom of foreign body in child is :
A. Cough B. Wheezing
C. Vomiting D. Dyspnoea

478. All of the following are associated with pulmonary hypoplasia except :
A. Diaphragmatic hernia
B. Asphyxiating thoracic malformation
C. Oligohydramnios
D. Air leak syndrome

479. Postural stridor with dysphagia in an infant is usually caused by :
A. Laryngomalacia
B. Aberrant vessels
C. Acute largngotracheo-bronchitis
D. TB in upper airways

480. Inhalation of 100% oxygen results in disappearance of central cyanosis in all of the following conditions, except :
A. Tetralogy of Fallot
B. Diffuse interstiital fibrosis
C. Chronic obstructive lung disease
D. Status asthmaticus

481. Stridor due to supraglottic obstruction differs from tracheal obstruction by following except :
A. Less serious B. Cry muffled
C, Dyspnoea more marked D. Cough less marked

482. In children above 6 years, ASOM is most often caused by :
A. H. influenzae B. Pneumococci
C. Staph. albus D. Aspergillus

483. Regarding staph. pneumonia, all are true except :
A. Lobar in distribution B. Hilar lymphadenopathy
C. Pneumatococle D. Pleural involvement

484. Patient with bronchiectasis may give a past history of :
A. Chickenpox B. Mumps
C. Whooping cough D. Typhoid

485. Alveolar-arterial tension gradient increases in all except :
A. Diffusion defects
B. Hypoventilation
C. R—> L shunt
D. Ventilation perfusion abnormality

Ans.	477. B	478. A	479. A	480. A	481. C	482. B
	483.B	484. C	485. B			

486. A patients with blood chemistry of pH 7.3, PCO2-65 mm, PO2< 40 mm. Diagnosis is :

A. COPD
B. ARDS (Acute Resp. distress Syndrome)
C. TOF (Tetralogy of Fallot)
D. None of the above

487. Lung abscess is caused by following except :

A. Staphylococcus B. Pneumococci
C. Klebsiella D. E. histolytica

488. Acute bronchiolitis is characterized by following except :

A. Caused by respiratory syncytial virus
B. Cough is infrequent
C. Expiratory dyspnoea
D. In earlier life leads to bronchial asthma
E. Humidified oxygen is used for treatment

489. The commonest presentation of miliary tuberculosis is :

A. Fever B. Weight loss
C. Dyspnoea D. Chest pain

490. Negative Mantoux test is important in :

A. Pulmonary Koch's B. Sarcoidosis
C. Carcinoma bronchus D. Lymphoma

491. Creaky or croupy cough is heard in :

A. Foreign body inhalation B. Bronchiolitis
C. Asthma D. Tracheitis

492. Which of the following viral infection in childhood is associated with bronchiectasis :

A. Mumps B. Measles
C. Rhinovirus D. Chicken pox

493. Which one of the following is true of Transient Tachypnoea of Newborn (TTNB) ?

A. It is the commonest respiratory disorder caused by absence of surfactant
B. In premature babies, it is often fatal
C. Onset of respiratory distress is immediately after birth and it rarely lasts beyond 48 hours
D. It often leads to chronic lung disease

494. Tidal volume in a 3 Kg infant with respiratory rate of 28 per min is about :

A. 10 ml B. 16 ml
C. 25 ml D. 50 ml

Ans.	486. A	487. D	488. B	489. A	490. A	491. D
	492. B	493. C	494. B			

495. Hyaline membrane seen in the lung is composed of :

A. Globulin B. Albumin
C. Mucoprotein D. Polysaccharide

496. Surfactant precursors appear as inclusion bodies in alveolar lining cells by ———— weeks :

A. 20 B. 24
C. 28 D. 32

497. Mediastinal widening is found in :

A. Histiocytic lymphoma B. Prolymphatic leukemias
C. CML with blast crisis D. T cell ALL

498. Transient tachypnoea of new born, following are true except :

A. Mild pleural effusion
B. Air bronchogram
C. Reticular shadow
D. Prominent interlobular fissure

499. Ghon's focus is :

A. Primary complex of TB B. Post primary TB
C. Miliary TB D. TB lymph nodes

500. Grunting respiration in the new born is suggestive of :

A. Congestive cardiac failure B. Respiratory disease
C. Acidosis D. Choanal atresia

501. Most common cause of Acute coryza :

A. Rhinovirus B. RSV
C. Influenza virus D. Corona virus

W502. Tuberculous pleural effusion is characterized by all except :

A. Haemorrhagic B. LDH more than 60%
C. ↑ mesothelial cells D. Deaminase

503. Low glucose in pleural effusion is seen in all except :

A. Rheumatoid arthritis B. Empyema
C. Malignant pleural effusion D. Dressler's syndrome

504. Bronchial obstruction in children with asthma is due to :
Consider the following causes :

I. Mucosal oedema
II. Increased secretions
III. Smooth muscle spasm
IV. Mucosal necrosis

A. I, II and III B. I and III
C. II and IV D. I, II, III and IV

Ans.					
495. B	**496. B**	**497. D**	**498. B**	**499. A**	**500. B**
501. A	**502. NONE**	**503. D**	**504. A**		

505. Which is not a feature of childhood asthma :

A. Raised IgE levels
B. History of atopic dermatitis
C. Absence of wheezing after exercise
D. Improves with age

506. A 7-month old infant has been hospitalised with respiratory distress, fever and minimal lung signs. The X-ray chest reveals hyperlucency Blood count is normal. The most likely diagnosis is :

A. Bronchopneumonia   B. Bronchiolitis
C. Collapse of the lung   D. Foreign body

507. In a child suffering from penumonia with rapid deterioration of clinical conditon, pneumatoceles, and pleural effusion on roentgenogram, the causative organisms besides staphylococcus aureus would include all of the following except :

A. Klebsiella   B. H. influenzae
C. E. coli   D. Strept. pneumoniae

508. The first drug for a child with evidence of severe bronchospasm in anaphylaxis is :

A. Oral prednisolone   B. I.V. Aminophylline
C. S.C. Adrenaline   D. I.M. Deriphylline

509. All of the following occur in acute resp. distress syndrome is all except :

A. Anemia
B. Groundglass appearance on X-ray
C. L : S ratio below one associated with severe RDS
D. Cyanosis

510. Erythromycin is the drug of choice in the treatment of childhood infection due to the following organisms, except :

A. Pertusis   B. Mycoplasma pneumoniae
C. Pneumocystis carinii   D. Chlamydia trachomatis

511. All of the following are beneficial in the management of acute attacks of bronchial asthma in children, except :

A. High concentration of humidified oxygen
B. Salbutamol nebuliser
C. Intravenous hydrocortisone
D. Sodium cromoglycate nebuliser

512. Lung abscesses in children may be produced by ll of the following organisms, except :

A. Pneumococcus   B. Entamoeba histolytica
C. Klebsiella pneumoniae   D. Staphylococcus aureus

Ans.	**505. C**	**506. B**	**507. C**	**508. C**	**509. A**	**510. C**
	511. D	**512. B**				

513. Unilateral blood stained nasal discharge in a 6 years old boy is commonly due to :

A. Enlarged adenoids
B. Chronic maxillary sinusitis
C. Foreign body in nostril
D. Choanal atresia

514. The sequential changes in acute bronchiolitis are as follows :

A. Dyspnoea, Resp. Acidosis, Resp. Alkalosis, Metabolic Acidosis
B. Resp. Acidosis, Metabolic Acidosis, Resp. Alkalosis, Dyspnoea
C. Metabolic acidosis, Dyspnoea, Resp. Alkalosis, Metabolic Acidosis
D. Dyspnoea, Resp. Alkalosis, Resp. Acidosis, Metabolic Acidosis.

515. In a child caesation of breathing for 20 sec. with bradycardia is :

A. Apnea
B. Dyspnea
C. Cheyne Stokes respiratio
D. None

516. Break down after breath holding is due to :

A. J-receptors
B. Increased PCO2 level
C. Fatigue of intricatory muscles
D. Elastic recoil of diaphragm/lungs

517. Child's respiratory physiology differs from adult because of :

A. Smaller airways
B. Increased O2 demand
C. Decreased tidal volume
D. Decreased residual volume

518. True about transient tachypnoea of the newborn is :

A. Air bronchogram seen
B. Common in preterm infants
C. Interlobar fissure effusion
D. Respiratory distress resolves in 6-10 days

519. An infant presents with clinical evidence of pneumonia which is confirmed with roentgeno-graph.The child deteriorates further and roentgenogram taken 12 hours later shows pleural effusion.The most likely cause of pneumonia is:

A. H.influenzae
B. Klebsiella
C. Pneumococcus
D. Staphylococcus

520. In obstructive lung disease all the following pulmonary functiopn test values are decreased except:

A. Forced vital capacity (FVC)
B. Forced expiratory volume in 1 sec. as per cent of FVC
C. Forced expiratory flow from 20 to 75% of FVC
D. Residual volume

Ans.	513. C	514. D	515. A	516. A	517. A	518. C
	519. C	520. D				

521. Match List-I (Conditions) with List-II (Findings) and select the correct answer using the codes given below the Lists:

List-I	List-II
A. Transient tachypnoea of the newborn	1. Incidence is reduced by good suctioning of oropharynx after head is delivered
B. Respiratory distress syndrome	2. Often seen following caesarean section
C. Bronchopulmonary dysplasia	3. May occur following trauma to chest during delivery
D. Meconium aspiration syndrome	4. Hyperexpansion with focal hyperlucency alternating with strands of opacification in chest radiograph
	5 In preterms with surfactant deficiency

Codes:

	a	b	c	d
A.	3	4	2	1
B.	2	5	4	1
C.	5	2	4	3
D.	2	5	1	3

522. Acidemia is usually manifested clinically by :

A. Kussmaul's breathing B. Sunken, soft eyeballs
C. Both D. Neither

523. Digital clubbing is not found in a child with which of the following :

A. Asthma
B. Bronchiectasis
C. Cyanotic congenital heart disease
D. Lung abscess

524. The following is contraindicated in the management of bronchiolitis :

A. The child should be nursed in a humid atmosphere
B. Adequate sedation should be given to prevent the child crying and exerting himself
C. It is important to ensure adequte hydration
D. There is no convincing evidence of the role of steroids in the management of bronchiolitis

Ans.	521. B	522. A	523. A	524. B

525. The most common cause of cor pulmonale in children is :

A. Bronchopneumonia B. Cystic fibrosis
C. Scoliosis D. None of the above

526. Epiglottitis is commonly treated with :

A. Tracheostomy
B. High environemental humidity
C. Early antimicrobial therapy
D. All of the above

527. Drug of choice for a child with pneumococcal pneumonia is :

A. Streptomycin B. Erythromycin
C. Chloromycetin D. Penicillin

528. Spasmodic croup most commonly occurs in ages of :

A. 1-3 months B. 6-9 months
C. 1-3 years D. 3-5 years

529. Which dose of adrenaline would be most appropriate for a 6 years old child with asthma ?

A. 0.1 ml (1 : 1000 solution) B. 0.5 ml (1 : 1000 solution)
C. 1.5 ml (1 : 1000 solution) D. 2.0 ml (1 : 1000 solution)

530. In case there is induction of premature labor, which of the following drug is useful in preventing hyaline membrane disease ?

A. Hydrocortisone B. Indomethacin
C. Propranolol D. Salbutamol

531. A child presents with hoarseness of voice, croupy cough and asthmatic wheeze. Most probable diagnosis is :

A. Asthmatic bronchitis
B. Bronchopneumonia
C. Retropharyngeal abscesshai
D. Foreign body in larynx

532. Intrathoracic primary tuberculosis is difficult to differentiate in X-ray from :

A. Carcinoma B. Sarcoidosis
C. Bronchopneumonia D. Ascariasis

533. Congenital pulmonary sequestrations are best diagnosed by :

A. Tomograms B. Fluoroscopy
C. Bronchograms D. Aortography

534. Weakness and paralysis of external muscles of respiration is found most frequently in infants with :

A. Amyotonia congenita B. Pneumothorax
C. Poliomyelitis D. Bronchopneumonia

Ans.	525. B	526. D	527. D	528. C	529. A	530. A
	531. D	532. B	533. D	534. A		

535. **In a 1 years old child, during true allergic asthmatic paroxysms, the X-ray signs resemble :**
A. Bilateral atelectasis
B. Bilateral obstructive emphysema
C. Bilateral pneumonia
D. Bilateral pnuemothorax

536. **A 2-year old healthy child suddenly develops breathlessness while playing. What is the most likely cause?**
A. Status asthmaticus
B. Pneumothorax
C. Foreign body aspiration
D. Cardiac failure

537. **The main aim of Tuberculosis treatment is :**
A. Bacteriological cure
B. Radiological cure
C. To prevent complications
D. Contact tracing

538. **All the following are true regarding reactions following BCG vaccination except :**
A. Maximum size of papule is reached at 5 weeks
B. Heals within 6-12 weeks
C. Ulceration with crust
D. Suppurative lymphadenitis

539. **According to WHO, TB is controlled when the prevalence among below 14 years of age is :**
A. Below 1% B. 5%
C. 1% D. 10%

540. **The best single laboratory aid in the diagnosis of tuberculosis is :**
A. Sputum examination B. Chest X-ray
C. Skin test D. Physical examination

541. **According to WHO, the point of control of Tuberculosis is prevalence less than ——— % tuberculin positivity among children in age- group ——— years :**
A. 1,0-12 B. 1,0-14
C. 0.5, 0-12 D. 0.5-1-12

542. **Overall average prevalence of infection of tuberculosis is ——— % :**
A. 20 B. 25
C. 30 D. 40

Ans.	535. B	536.C	537.A	538.D	539.A	540.A
	541. B	542. C				

543. The direct BCG vaccination in India is given upto age of

A. 10 year B. 15 year
C. 20 year D. 25 year

544. Mantoux test is read after ——— hours but before ———hours :

A. 24, 72 B. 48, 72
C. 72, 96 D. 72, 120

545. 0.1 ml of BCG contains ——— mg moist weight :

A. 0.050 B. 0.025
C. 0.075 D. 0.100

546. A positive Mantoux test indicates that the child :

A. Is suffering from active TB
B. Has had BCG vaccination recently
C. Has had tuberculosis infection
D. All of the above

547. Tuberculin test true is :

A. Induration more than 10 mm in 72 hours
B. Measure incidence of disease
C. Used for diagnosis of TB
D. Measure immunity

548. Tuberculin unit is :

A. 1 unit of PPD RT23 B. 0.000001 unit of PPD RT 23
C. 0.1 C.C. of BCG D. I.C.C. of PPD RT 23

549. Tubercular bacilli are maximally seen in :

A. Lymphnode B. Cavity
C. Lymph vessels D. Blood

550. Diluent for BCG vaccine is :

A. Distilled water B. Normal saline
C. Dextrose D. KOH

551. Best treatment of tuberculosis is :

A. Case finding and treatment
B. BCG
C. Free drugs
D. Good diet

552. A poor woman with active tuberculosis is breast feeding a newborn. Best management is :

A. Stop breast feeding
B. Start antitubercular drugs is mother
C. Give INH to newborn
D. Give INH + BCG to newborn

Ans.	543. C	544. B	545. C	546. D	547. A	548. A
	549. B	550. B	551. A	552. D		

553. A Mantoux test is considered positive when the induration at the site of injection of ITU of PPD read after 72 hrs is :

A. 10 mm or more
B. 6-9 mm
C. 3-5 mm
D. None of the above

554. Which of the following is the most frequent extra pulmonic site for tuberculosis ?

A. Pericardium
B. Kidney
C. Peritoneum
D. Lymph nodes

555. The primary mode of transmission of tuberculosis is :

A. Fomites
B. Airborne
C. Arthropods
D. Files

556. Prevalence of tubercular infection is best assessed by :

A. Tuberculin test
B. Chest X-ray
C. Sputum for AFB culture
D. Microscopy of sputum for AFB

557. For tuberculous patients who can attend a hospital or health centre, the following combination has been recommended bi-weekly :

A. Streptomycin-1 gm + INH-900 mg+ Pyridoxine-30 mg
B. Streptomycin-1 gm+INH-650mg + Pyridoxine - 10 mg
C. Streptomycin -0.75 gm+INH-450 mg+ Pyridoxine -10mg
D. Streptomycin-1 gm+INH-1gm + Pyridoxine 100 mg

558. BCG vaccine once prepared should be used within :

A. 1 day
B. 2 days
C. 3 days
D. 4 days

559. Which of the following is not a feature of miliary tuberculosis :

A. Mantoux test is usually negative
B. Meningitis is a usual complication
C. Dyspnoea is a usual presentation
D. Septicemia is rare

560. Positive tuberculin test in a child below 2 years indictes :

A. High susceptibility to tuberculosis
B. Active tuberculosis
C. An allergic reaction to tuberculosis
D. Resistance to tuberculosis

561. Tuberculin sensitivity was done by using PPD tuberculin. The dosage was :

A. 1 TU
B. 2 TU
C. 5 TU
D. 10 TU

562. Assessment of magnitude of T.B. & its trend in community is by :

A. Tuberculin Conversion Index
B. Incidence Rate
C. Prevatenc Rate
D. Fatality Rate

Ans.	553. A	554. D	555. B	556. A	557. B	558. A
	559. B	560. B	561. A	562. A		

563. Following is true of T.B.

A. > 104 organisms req. in sputum for detection
B. Mantoux test is often negative in early stages
C. Monotherapy is best
D. Treatment given for 2 years

564. Not true about tuberculin test :

A. Specific
B. >10 mm
C. Absence of reaction should be interpreted cautiously
D. INH convertes + to negative

565. True about Mantoux test is :

A. Test is read before 48 hours
B. Those with 6-9 mm induration have more chances of developing TB
C. Majority of new caes occur in tuberculin negative person
D. Induration > 10 mm is positive

566. In milliary TB following are seen, except :

A. Chest sign may be -ve
B. Multiple crypts may be seen
C. Pulmonary form may mimic acute bronchiotitis
D. Temperature may be subnormal

567. 'DOTS' is :

A. Short term chemotherapy under direct observation
B. Long term chemotherapy under direct observation
C. Long term chemotherapy without supervision
D. Free drug distribution to poor patients

568. Positive Mantoux means induration :

A. 2 mm in transverse direction
B. 2 mm is Horizontal direction
C. 5-9 mm Diameter
D. > 10 mm Diameter

569. Important measures to prevent drug resistance for tuberculosis include all of the folowingexcept:

A. Complete treatment with drug combinations
B. Using drugs to which bacterial sensitivity is reported in the community
C. Prompt defaulter action
D. Pre-treatment sputum culture and sensitivity of cases

570. Paucibacillary, single lesion, single dose Rx is :

A. Rif, oflox, clarithromycin B. Dapsone, Rif., clofazimine
C. Rif., oflox, minocycline D. Dapsone, clofazimine

Ans.	563. A	564. A	565. D	566. D	567. A	568. D
	569. D	570. D				

571. MC cause for drug resistance in TB in India :

A. INH
B. Rifampin
C. Streptomycin
D. Ethambutol

572. False about DOTS is :

A. Continuation phase drugs are given in a multiblister pack
B. Medication is to be taken in presence of a health worker
C. Biweekly dosage
D. Improves compliance

573. Which of the following is true about tuberculin test :

A. It gives the immune status of patient
B. It may be negative in dissociated tuberculosis
C. It tells about prior exposure to Mycobacterium tuberculosis only
D. It is highly positive in a post measles case

574. Prevalence of Tuberculosis infection is measured by :

A. Tuberculin Test
B. Chest X-ray
C. Sputum microscopy for AFB
D. Sputum culture for AFB

575. Of the following, which is incorrect about BCG scar formation?

A. Size is 4-8 mm in 5 weeks
B. Papule forms within a week
C. Shallow ulcer with crust
D. Spontaenous healing within 6-12 weeks

576. A person with tuberculosis on domiciliary Treatment is expected to do all except :

A. Collect drugs regularly
B. Dispose sputum safely
C. Use separate vessels
D. Report to PMC if new symptom arises

577. Each of the following structures is found in the posterior mediastinum except :

A. Azygos vein
B. Descending aorta
C. Phrenic nerve
D. Vagus nerve

578. Each of the upper nine intercostal spaces has the following combination of intercostal arteries :

A. One posterior and one anterior
B. One posterior and two anterior
C. Two posterior and one anterior
D. Two posterior and two anterior

Ans.	571. A	572. C	573. B	574. A	575. B	576. C
	577. C	578. D				

579. Each of the following has an attachment to scapula except :

A. Pectoralis major B. Pectoralis minor
C. Biceps brachii D. Triceps

580. Which of the following events does not take place at the level of the sternal angle ?

A. The arch of the aorta begins
B. The azygos vein joins the superior vena cava
C. The superior vena cava joins the right atrium
D. The trachea bifurcates

581. Which of the following is most anterior in thoracic inlet

A. Sternohyoid B. Brachiocebhalic vein
C. Common carotid artery D. Subclavian artery

582. The following structures form the boundaries to the superior entrance into the axilla except the :

A. Clavicle B. Coracoid process
C. Upper border of scapula D. Outer border of first rib

583. Costal margin of 3-5 ribs only give origin to :

A. Pectoralis major B. Pectoralis minor
C. Subclavius D. Serratus anterior

584. The blood vessel that does not take part in supplying the oesophagus is the :

A. Aortic B. Gastric
C. Inferior phrenic D. Internal mammary

585. The oesophgus commences at the following level :

A. Lower end of cricoid B. C5 vertebra
C. 10 cm from incisor teeth D. C7 vertebra

586. Attachments to first rib are following except :

A. Scalene anterior B. Scalene medius
C. Scalene posterior D. Suprapleural membrane

587. Oesophagus crosses the diaphragm at level of :

A. T8 B. T10
C. T12 D. L2

588. 'J' receptiors are situated in :

A. Heart B. Blood vessels
C. Alveolar interstitium D. Carotid body

589. Diaphragm is at lowest level in which position :

A. Standing B. Supine
C. Prone D. Sitting

Ans.	579. A	580. B	581. B	582. C	583. C	584. A
	585. C	586. A	587. A	588. C	589. A	

590. Structure affected first when accessory cervical rib is stretched :
A. Lat. cord of brachial plexus
B. Medial cord of brachial plexus
C. Vessel involvement
D. Small muscle wasting of hand

591. Anastomosis freely occurs between :
A. Coronary arteries
B. Cerebral arteries
C. Bronchial & pulmonary arteries
D. Splenic arteries

592. Following muscles cause retraction of shoulder except :
A. Trapezius B. Serratus anterior
C. Rhomboid major D. Rhomboid minor

593. Thoracic duct is also called :
A. Hensen's duct B. Bernard's duct
C. Pecquet duct D. Hoffman's duct

594. Xiphisternal junction is usually at the level of disc between the following thoracic vertebrae :
A. 9 and 10 B. 8 and 7
C. 1 and 12 D. None

595. The —— vein connects the lateral thorcic vein cranially with the superfical epigastric vein caudally :
A. Internal thoracic B. Musculophrenic
C. Thoracoepigastric D. Anterior mediastinal

596. The internal thoracic veins are tributaries of the :
A. Azygos B. Subclavian
C. Internal jugular D. Brachiocephalic

597. The length of oesophagus (in inches) is :
A. 5 B. 8
C. 10 D. 15

598. Arterial supply of second intercostal space is by :
A. Deep cervical B. Superior intercostal
C. Musculophrenic D. Posterior intercostal

599. The contents of the superior mediastinum are the following except :
A. Inferior vena cava B. Arch of aorta
C. Thoracic duct D. Right common carotid artery

600. All of the following muscle originate in the scapula except :
A. Deltoid B. Teres major
C. Coracobrachialis D. Trapezius

Ans.	590. B	591. C	592. B	593. C	594. A	595. C
	596. D	597. C	598. D	599. A	600. D	

601. **Motor supply of the diaphragm :**
A. Thoracodorsal B. Intercostal nerves
C. Phrenic nerve D. Sympathetic

602. **Ventral ramus of second thoracic nerve gives rise to the :**
A. Median nerve B. Lateral pectoral nerve
C. Intercostobrachial nerve D. Radial nerve

603. **The chief pathway of the lymph vessels of thorax is the :**
A. Thoracic duct
B. Intercostal lymph trunks
C. Bronchomediastinal lymph trunk
D. Right jugular trunk

604. **Esophagus starts at :**
A. Posterior to cricoid B. Posterior to trachea
C. Posterior to thyroid D. Posterior to glotti

605. **Left superior intercostal vein drains into :**
A. Azygos vein B. Left innominate vein
C. Hemiazygos vein D. Internal thoracic vein

606. **Direct extension of the aortic plexus below the aortic bifurcation is the :**
A. Pudendal nerve B. Presacral nerve
C. Sympathetic trunk D. Hypogastric nerve

607. **The ligamentum arteriosum connects arch of aorta with :**
A. Pulmonary trunk
B. Superior vena cava
C. Left branch of pulmonary artery
D. Subclavian artery

608. **The thoracic duct open at the junction of :**
A. Rt. Internal jugular and right subclavian
B. Two branchiocephlaic veins
C. Left internal jugular and left subclavian
D. None of the above

609. **The girdle of upper limb is constituted by the :**
A. Scapula B. Clavicle
C. Humerus D. A and C only

610. **Lattisimus dorsi is supplied by nerve :**
A. Thoracodorsal B. Axillary
C. Long thoracic D. Musculocutaneous

611. **Which of the following heart chamber is closely related to oesophagus :**
A. Left atrium B. Right atrium
C. Right ventricle D. Left ventricle

Ans.	601. C	602. C	603. C	604. A	605. B	606. B
	607. B	608. C	609. D	610. A	611. A	

612. The contents of middle mediastinum are all except :

A. Ascending aorta B. Trunk of pulmonary artery
C. Arch of Azygous vein D. None of the above

613. Which of the following does not pass through diaphragm :

A. Inferior vena cava B. Aorta
C. Oesophagus D. None of the above

614. Thoracic duct crosses from right to the left at the level of :

A. T_1 B. T_4
C. T_6 D. T_8

615. In a cross section of thorax at T4, which is found :

A. Azygos vein B. Right brachiocephalic vein
C. Thoracic duct D. L. subclavian artery

616. The superior most opening in the diaphragm is :

A. Aortic B. Vena caval
C. Oesophagea D. Lateral arcuate foramen

617. Oesophgeal constrictions are at the following sites except :

A. Tracheal bifurcation B. Aortic arch
C. Passage through diaphragm D. None of the above

618. Clavipectoral fascia is pierced by all of the following except :

A. Thoracocrominal artery B. Axillary vein
C. Cephalic vein D. Lateral pectoral nerve

619. Which of the following is related to anterior surface of scalenus anterior except :

A. Subclavian artery B. Subclavian vein
C. Phrenic nerve D. Transverse cervical

620. Thoracic sympathetic chain is situated :

A. Near heads of 2-10 ribs
B. Infront of posterior inter costal vessels
C. Infront of vertebral column
D. Passes superficial arcuate ligament

621. All of the following are tributaries of Azygous vein except :

A. Left posterior intercostal veins
B. Hemiazygous vein
C. Right posterior intercostal veins
D. Right bronchal vein

622. Nucleus thoracic is represented in medulla oblongata as :

A. Nucleus cuneatus B. Nucleus gracilis
C. Inferior olivary nucleus D. Accessory cuneatus nucleus

623. The terminal branches of internal mammary artery are :

A. Right gastroepiploic
B. Superior epigastric

Ans.	612. D	613. D	614. B	615. A	616. B	617. D
	618. B	619. A	620. D	621. A	622. D	623. B

C. Left anterior descending artery
D. Superior pancreatioduodenal

624. Which of the following structures lies deep to the fourth intercostal space on the right side of sternum ?
A. Brachiocephalic artery B. Left brachiocephalic vein
C. Right brachiocephalic vein D. Right atrium

625. Azygos vein enters thorax through which of the following openings of diaphragm :
A. Medial arcuate foramen B. Inferior vena cava
C. Aortic D. Oesophageal

626. Following glands are found in oesophagus :
A. Tyson's glands B. Weber's glands
C. Brunner's glands D. Cobelli's glands

627. Central tendon of Diaphragm is developed from :
A. Septum transversu B. Pleuroperitoneal membrane
C. Dossal mesentry D. Dorsal thoracic wall

628. A typical intercostal nerve supplies :
A. Skin only
B. Skin & intercostal muscles
C. Skin, intercostal muscles & pleura
D. None of the above

629. The most important component of the development of diaphragm is :
A. Pleuroperitoneal canal B. Septum transverum
C. Shelf from body wall D. None of the above

630. In thoracic esophagus, following are true except:
A. Circular layer
B. Longitudinal muscles
C. It is laterally flattened
D. Pharyngooesophageal junction is narrowest part

631. About thoracolumbar facia all are true except :
A. Gives attachment to transversus abdominis & int. oblique medially
B. Attached to the tip of spine
C. Attached to tip of transverse process
D. Lies posterior to post abd. muscles

632. Membrana tectoria is an upward projection of :
A. Inter longitudinal ligament
B. Posterior longitudinal ligament
C. Alar ligament
D. Apical ligament

Ans.	624. D	625. C	626. D	627. A	628. B	629. B
	630. C	631. D	632. B			

633. All the following muscles are involved in forced inspiration except :

A. Diaphragm B. Pectoralis minor
C. Sternomastoid muscle D. Lattisimuss Dorsi

634. At the midaxillary line, parietal pleura extends upto the level of :

A. 8th rib B. 9th rib
C. 10th rib D. 11th rib

635. Hilum of right lung is arched by :

A. Recurrent laryngeal nerve B. Azygos vein
C. Thoracic duct D. Sup. vena cava

636. Bronchopulmonary segment contains all the following except :

A. Independent pulmonary artery
B. Independant pulmonary vein
C. Teriary bronchiole
D. Conical segiment

637. Rt middle lobe consists of which bronchopulmonary segment :

A. Superior & inferior B. Medical and lateral
C. Anterior and posterior D. Apical and lateral

W.638. Parts of left lower lobe of lung except :

A. Apical B. Ant. basal
C. Post. basal D. Medial basal

639. In midclavicular line costo diaphragmatic line of pleural reflection is at :

A. 6th rib B. 8th rib
C. 10th rib D. 12th rib

640. Sequestration of lung is seen in :

A. Right upper lobe B. Right lower lobe
C. Lateral basal D. Posterior part of left lung

641. The arteries supplying the pleura are the following except :

A. Bronchial B. Pericardio phrenic
C. Posterior intercostal D. Internal mammary

642. Consider the following statements regarding bronchopulmonary segments :

1. The middle lobe of the right lung has medial and lateral segments
2. The medial basal segment may be absent on the left side
3. Some diseases may be localised to one segment
4. Surgical removal of a segment possible

Of these statements

A. 1,2 and 3 are correct
B. 1 and 3 are correct
C. 2 and 4 are correct
D. 1,2,3 and 4 are correct

Ans.	**633. D**	**634. C**	**635. B**	**636. B**	**637. B**
	638. NONE	**639. B**	**640. D**	**641. B**	**642. D**

643. Nerves to the pulmoanry pleura come from :

A. Vagus
B. Phrenic
C. Intercostal
D. All of the above

644. Bronchopulmonary segment is a unit in the architecture of the lung. The best guide to the intersegmental planes would be the :

A. Segmental bronchi
B. Branches of the segmental artery
C. Veins draining the segment
D. Connective tissue septa

645. A rare abnormality sometimes occurs in right lung is called :

A. Thymic lobe
B. Azygos lobe
C. Caval lobe
D. Pulmonary lobe

646. The pyramid of lung supplied by each segmental bronchus constitutes :

A. A bronchial lobe
B. Pulmonary segment
C. A bronchopulmonary segment
D. An azygos lobe

647. The base of lung :

A. Is grooved by subclavian artery
B. Fills the cervical pleura
C. Is deeply concave
D. None of the above

648. The roots of lungs include the :

A. Lymphatics
B. Bronchi
C. Pulmnary and bronchial vessels
D. All of the above

649. The strongest part of the parietal pleura is the :

A. Costal
B. Pulmonary
C. Mediastinal
D. Diaphragmatic

650. Which of the following are the characteristics of pulmonary parenchyma

1. It receives its oxygenated arterial supply via the branches of the thoracic aorta
2. It has no lymph drainage
3. It has venous drainage into the azygos system of veins
4. It has ciliated columnar epithelial lining throughout

Select the correct answer using the codes given below :

Code :

A. 1, 2 and 3
B. 1 and 3
C. 2 and 4
D. 1,2,3 and 4

Ans.	**643. D**	**644. C**	**645. A**	**646. C**	**647. C**	**648. D**
	649. A	**650. B**				

651. The weight of the right lung of a healthy adult is approximately :

A. 400 gms B. 480 gms

C. 620 gm D. 800 gms

652. The weight of the left lung of a healthy adult is approximately :

A. 250 gms B. 450 gms

C. 570 gms D. 730 gms

653. Consider the following structures of the root of the right lung :

1. Lower pulmonary vein
2. Right principal bronchus
3. Superior lobe bronchus
4. Pulmonary artery

The correct sequence in the order from above downwards, of these structures comprising the root of the right lung is :

A. 4,3,2,1 B. 4,3,1,2

C. 3,4,2,1 D. 3,4,1,2

654. The phrenic nerves transmit sensory fiberes from :

A. Pericardium B. Liver

C. Inferior vena cava D. All of these

655. To pass a needle into the pleural cavity, the following strucutes will have to be pierced in the midaxillary line, except :

A. Internal intercosatal muscle B. Levator costarum

C. Parietal pleura D. Tranversus thoracis

656. All of the following are cells of bronchial epithelium except :

A. Clara cells B. Kulchitsky cells

C. Goblet cells D. Globule Leucocytes

657. The functional tissue of lungs is :

A. Alveoli B. Bronchi

C. Resp. bronchiole D. Terminal bronchiole

658. Which of the following structure is not situated between the neck of the first rib and apex of the lung ?

A. First posterior intercostal vein

B. Superior intercostal artery

C. Thoracic duct

D. Sympathetic trunk

659. What is the correct sequence of the following groups of lymph nodes through which lymph from the lung passes ?

1. Tracheobranchial nodes
2. Bronchopulmonary nodes
3. Bronchomediastinal nodes

Ans.	651. C	652. C	653. C	654. D	655. B	656. D
	657. A	658. C	659. D			

Select the correct answer using the codes given below :

Codes :

A. 1,3,2 B. 3,2,1

C. 2,3,1 D. 2,1,3

660. Pulmonary vein (2-4 in number) drain into :

A. Right atrium

B. Right ventricle

C. Superiorly on the posterior surface of left atrium

D. Interiorly on posterior surface of left atrium

661. The blood supply of lung tissue is :

A. Pulm. veins B. Pulm. arteries

C. Bronchial arteries D. Lower thoracic aorta

662. Impressions on the surface of right lung are made by all except :

A. Azygous vein B. Superior vena cava

C. Aortic arch D. Right brachiocephalic vein

663. Consider the following statements :

Development of lung tissue medial to the right common cardinal veins results in :

1. Accessory lobe
2. Azygos lobe
3. Lobe of azygos vein

Of these statements

A. 1,2 and 3 are correct B. 1 and 2 are correct

C. 2 and 3 are correct D. 1 and 3 are correct

664. Below the root of lung, double layer of mediastinal pleura that is directed caudally and medially is :

A. Cupola B. Hilus

C. Pulmonary ligament D. Mediastinal fascia

665. Most interior structure of hilum of the lung includes :

A. Superior pulmonary vein B. Inferior pulmonary vein

C. Bronchus D. Pulmonary artery

666. Lingula is a part of :

A. Left upper lobe B. Left lower lobe

C. Right upper lobe D. Right middle lobe

667. The following are the true respiratory movements except :

A. Rotation at sternal end

B. Elevation of ribs

C. Pump handle movement of sternum

D. Buckle handle movement of ribs

Ans.	660. C	661. C	662. C	663. D	664. C	665. B
	666. A	667. A				

668. The parietal pleura is supplied by all except :

A. Somatic nerves
B. Phrenic nerves
C. Intercostal nerve
D. None of the above

669. The lingula of the left lung :

A. Is above the cardiac notch
B. Is a part of the lower lober
C. Has a superior and inferior broncho-pulmonary segments
D. Corresponds to the lobe of azygos vein of right lung

670. Sequestrated lung is supplied most commonly by :

A. Bronchial arteries
B. Descending aorta
C. Subclavian artery
D. Costal arteries

671. Intercostobrachial N is a branch of :

A. I intercostal N
B. II intercostal N
C. III intercostal N
D. Upper trunk of Brachial plexus

672. A common site of peanut lodgement in lungs is :

A. Rt Superior lobe bronchus
B. Trachea
C. Rt lower lobe bronchus
D. Left lower lobe bronchus

673. The most dependent part of the lung in the supine position :

A. Upper apical
B. Lower apical
C. Basal
D. Upper anterior

674. In the bronchial lining epithelium, one would find :

A. Clara cell, goblet cell, brush cell and Kulchitsky cell
B. Serous cell, goblet cell, clara cell and brush cell
C. Non-cilated cell, serous cell, basal cell and brush cell
D. Ciliated cell, goblet cell, basal cell and brush cell

675. True about phrenic nerve:

A. Arises from dorsal root of C3,4,5
B. Carries innervation from mediastinum and diaphragmatic surface of pleura and diaphragmatic peritoneum
C. Passes via left pleural cavity
D. It passes via caval opening

676. Discharge of tubercle bacilli in large numbers into the thoracic duct would most probably produce :

A. Pleural effusion
B. Miliary tuberculosis especially of lungs
C. Caseation of glands of neck
D. Severe military tuberculosis

677. Of the following pneumoconioses the one which is very often complicated by tuberculosis is :

A. Anthracosis
B. Berylliosis
C. Byssinosis
D. Silicosis
E. Siderosis

Ans.	668. D	669. D	670. B	671. B	672. A	673. B
	674. A	675. D	676. B	677. D		

678. Malignant tumur of the lung may be of any of the following types except :

A. Squamous cell carcinoma B. Anaplastic carcinoma
C. Clear cell carcinoma D. Adenocarcinoma
E. Epidermoid carcinoma

679. The commonest caviting secondaries in lungs is seen in :

A. Squamous cell carcinoma B. Adenocarcinoma
C. Seminoma testis D. Choriocarcinoma

680. Sequestration of lung is seen in :

A. Right upper lobe B. Right lower lobe
C. Lateral basal lobe D. Posterior part of left lung

681. Most pulmonary infarcts are :

A. White B. Asymptomatic
C. Secondary D. All of these
E. None of these

682. Cigarette smoking predisposes to which of the following lung cancer :

A. Adenocarcinoma B. Squamous cell carcinoma
C. Oat cell carcinoma D. b + c
E. All of the above

683. In compression atelectasis the collasped lung is nearest of the thoracic cage at :

A. Anterior wall B. Lateral wall
C. Posterior wall D. Upper pole
E. Lower pole

684. Gray hepatization of lungs is seen on day :

A. 1 B. 2—3
C. 3—5 D. 5—7

685. Which of the following tubercular focus in lungs is always apical :

A. Simon's focus B. Assman's focus
C. Aschoff Puhl focus D. Ghon's focus

686. The following is not a complication of tuberculosis :

A. Acute paraplegia B. Amyloidosis
C. Hypoplastic anaemia D. Cardiomyopathy

687. Which of the following primaries do not produce a smooth secondary in lungs :

A. Seminoma B. Carcinoma lymph node
C. Carcinoma thyroid D. Carcinoma lung

688. The type of emphysema most closely related to cigarette smoking is :

A. Focal B. Bullous
C. Centriacinar D. Panacinar

Ans.	678. C	679. A	680. D	681. C	682. D	683. C
	684. C	685. C	686. D	687. B	688. C	

689. Bronchogenic carcinoma may spread to the following except :

A. Liver B. Kidneys
C. Adrenal D. Gall Bladder

690. "Acinus" or "terminal respiratory unit" is the part of the lung :

A. Distal to the bifurcation of trachea
B. Distal to the proximal bronchiole
C. Distal to the terminal bronchiole
D. Distal to the alveolar duct

691. The minimum amount of air required to produce symptoms of air embolism is :

A. 10 ml B. 20 ml
C. 50 ml D. 100 ml

692. Pueumonia alba is caused by :

A. Streptoccus B. Pneumococcus
C. Mycobacteria D. Staphylococcus

693. Which of the following is not a histological type of carcinoma lung :

A. Small cell B. Oat cell
C. Squamous cell D. Transitional type

694. Petechiae on pleural and pericardial surface and squames in alveoli of an autopsied neonatal infant suggest :

A. A tranplacntally acquired viral infection
B. Intrauterine anoxia
C. A metaplastic epithelial response to oxygen therapy
D. A marked decrease in pulmonary surfactant
E. An inherent clotting defect

695. The most common termination of lobar pneumonia is :

A. Consolidation B. Resolution
C. Abscess formation D. Empyema

696. Pulmonary hypertension causes hypertrophy of the :

A. Right ventricle B. Left ventricle
C. Right atrium D. Left atrium

697. Lung autopsy in a neonate shows dark and firm lung. Some parts of the surface are depressed. Bubble like areas seen microscopically in the septa and alveoli. The findings are suggestive of :

A. Tricuspid atresia B. Pulmonary embolism
C. Hydrocephalus D. Atelectasis

Ans.	**689. D**	**690. C**	**691. D**	**692. C**	**693. D**	**694. B**
	695. B	**696. A**	**697. D**			

698. Acute massive collapse of lungs is a variety (or obstructive) atelectasis encountered in :

A. Bronchogenic carcinoma
B. Pulmonary lymhadenitis
C. Tuberculous meningitis
D. Abdominal surgery

699. The alveoli are filled with exudate; the air is displaced converting the lung into a solid organ. This description suggests :

A. Chronic bronchitis B. Bronchial asthma
C. Bronchiectasis D. Lobar pneumonia

700. The most common lung cancer as a consequence of asbestos exposure is :

A. Anaplastic Carcinoma B. Squanous cell carcinoma
C. Adenocarcinoma D. Sarcoma

701. Culture of pleural biopsy tissue is —— to culture of pleural fluid for demonstration of Mycobacterium TB :

A. Superior B. Inferior
C. Same D. Variable

702. Commonest type of bronchogenic carcinoma is :

A. Adenocarcinoma
B. Oat cell carcinoma
C. Squamous cell carcinoma
D. Large cell carcinoma

703. Mesothelioma of pleura is commonly associated with :

A. Asbestosis B. Anthracosis
C. Silicosis D. Siderosis

704. Sputum from an asthma patient may show :

A. Numerous eosinophils B. Curschmann's spirals
C. Charcot-Leyden crystals D. All of the above

705. Allergic bronchopulmonary aspergillosis is related to sarcoidosis involving the lung by which cell type?

A. Macrophage B. Plasma cell
C. Eosinophil D. Type II pneumocyte

706. All of the following clinical/pathological feature are characteristically seen in the adult respiratory distress syndrome (ARDS) except :

A. Heavy "meaty" lungs
B. Hyaline membrane formation
C. Hypoxaemia which does not respond to oxygen therapy
D. Proliferation of type 1 pneumocytes

Ans.	698. D	699. D	700. C	701. A	702. A	703. A
	704. D	705. C	706. D			

707. Brown induration of lung is seen in :

A. Silicosis
B. Siderosis
C. Asbestosis
D. Bagassosis

708. The commonest cause of hydropneumothorax in India is :

A. Bronchogenic carcinoma
B. Sarcoidosis
C. Emphysematous bulla rupture
D. Pulmonary Koch's

709. Venous congestion of lung, following is true :

A. Heart failure cells
B. Hypostalic pneumonia
C. Subcrepitant lungs
D. Fibrinous pleuresy

710. True about histological picture in viral pneumonia is all except :

A. Inflammatory reaction virtually localized to alveoli
B. Mononuclear inflammatory infilterate
C. Herpes simplex may cause bronchial wall hyperplasia
D. Superimposed bacterial infection

711. Multiple interstitial nodules are seen in :

A. Mitiary TB
B. Tropical eosinophitia
C. Lobar pneumonia
D. Abestosis

712. The diagnostic morphologic alteration in chronic bronchitis is :

A. Hyperplasia of bronchial muscus glands
B. Hypertrophy of smooth muscle
C. Presence of lymphoid follicles in bronchial wall
D. Metaplasia of lining epithelium

713. Commonest cells found in bronchoalveolar washings are :

A. Monocytes
B. Macrophages
C. Lymphages
D. Eosinophils

714. Most common form of TB in a child is :

A. Meningitis
B. Primary pulmonary tuberculosis
C. Primary pulmonary progressive TB
D. Adenopathy

715. Which is associated with Ca Lung :

A. Chromium
B. Berrylium
C. Asbestosis
D. Nickel

716. Commonest type of Emphysema is :

A. Panacinar
B. Centriacinar
C. Irregular
D. Obstructed

717. Surfactant in lung is produced by :

A. Type I cells
B. Type II cells
C. Kulchitsky's cells
D. Mast cells

Ans.					
707. B	708. C	709. C	710. C	711. D	712. A
713. B	714. C	715. C	716. B	717. B	

718. Tree bark like calcification in a Chest X-ray is suggestive of :

A. Artherosclerosis B. Syphilitic aneurysm
C. Neurofibromatosis D. Aorto-arteritis

719. The type of bronchogenic Ca with best prognosis is :

A. Oat cell B. Small cell
C. Large cell D. Squamous cell carcinoma

720. Alpha-I-antitrypsin deficiency occurs in :

A. Emphysema B. Bronchiectasis
C. Empyema D. Bronchogenic Ca

721. Paramalignant effusion is seen in :

A. Hypoproteinemia
B. Lymphatic block
C. Malignancy related cachexia
D. Bronchogenic carcinoma

722. Consider the following statements about Simon's focus :

1. It is component of primary complex
2. It is usually seen near the base of the lung
3. It is the result of haematogenous seeding during primary infection
4. Post-primary tuberculosis is caused in some cases by the spread of viable bacteria from Simon's focus

Of these statements :

A. 1,2 and 3 are correct B. 2 and 3 are correct
C. 1 and 4 are correct D. 3 and 4 are correct

723. Consider the following statements regarding tubercular infection in human beings :

1. In the case of tuberculosis, it is the dose of infection and not the virulence of the organism that determines whether the infection will be abortive or destructive
2. There is only racial resistance and no individual resistance to tuberculosis
3. Malnutrition is a contributory factor in the progression of tubercular infection
4. Rate of tubercular infection in adults is more amongst diabetics than amongst non-diabetics

Of these statements

A. 1,2,3 and 4 are correct B. 1 and 3 are correct
C. 2 and 4 are correct D. 3 and 4 are correct

724. Pleural effusion in cirrhosis is characterized by following except :

A. Pleural LDH > serum LDH B. Protein - 10 g/L
C. Glucose - 80 mg D. S.G. below 1.012

Ans. 718. B 719. D 720. A 721. B 722. D 723. D 724. B

725. Lung absces is common following —— pneumonia :
A. Streptococcal B. Staphylococcal
C. Viral D. Klebsiella

726. Primary infection with tuberculosis is most commonly characterized by :
A. Cavitary apical lesions
B. Multiple diffuse pulmonary calcifications
C. Peripheral lung lessions and regional lymph node involvement
D. Tuberculous pneumonia
E. Tuberculous meningitis

727. The lung carcinoma most common in non smokers is :
A. Sq. cell B. Large cell
C. Adenocarcinoma D. Small cell

728. In the stage of Gray hepatization :
A. WBC's fill the alveoli
B. RBC's fill the alveoli
C. Organisms fill the alveoli
D. Accumulation of fibrin

729. Filling of the alveoli with foamy, eosinophilic material, together with interstitial mononuclear infiltration, is most characteristic of pneumonia due to :
A. Staphylococcus B. Mycoplasma
C. Pneumococcus D. Pneumocystis

730. Hyaline membranes lining alveolar walls are a characteristic feature of :
A. Pulmonary proteniosis
B. Goodpasture's syndrome
C. Desquamative interstitial pneumonitis
D. Adult respiratory distress syndorme
E. Berylliosis

731. A man has Ca lung with nephrotic syndrome of type :
A. Mesangial type B. Minimal type
C. Membranous type D. Mesangio proliferative type

732. All of the following paraneoplastic syndromes are seen in Bronchogenic carcinoma except :
A. Myasesthenia gravis
B. Hypocalcemia
C. Hyperparathyroidism
D. Hypertrophic pulmonary osteoarthropathy

Ans. **725. B** **726. C** **727. C** **728. D** **729. D** **730. D** **731. C** **732. B**

733. The type of carcinoma arising from the scars of the lung :
A. Squamous cell carcinoma
B. Oat cell carcinoma
C. Adenocarcinoma
D. Undifferentiated carcinoma

734. The least common cause of calcification in the lung is :
A. Aspergillosis B. Tuberculosis
C. Histoplasmosis D. Amyloidosis

735. Characteristic sputum in bronchial asthma contains :
A. Curschmann's spirals B. Charcot-Leyden crystals
C. Eosinophils D. All of these

736. In amniotic fluid embolism the following are found in the maternal pulmonary microcirculation except :
A. Squamas from fetal skin
B. Lanugo hair
C. Fat from vernix caseosa
D. Myxoid tissue from umbilical cord

737. During the state of grey hepatisation in lobar pneumonia the alveoli are filled by :
A. Fibrin B. Organisms
C. RBC's D. WBC's

738. Lung is characterstically involved in :
A. Churg - Straus syndromeB. HSP
C. PAN D. ITP

739. Scar in lung tissue develops into :
A. Adenocarcinoma B. Oat cell Carcinoma
C. Squamous cell Carcinoma D. Columnar cell carcinoma

740. Characteristic of expectorant present in cryptogenic fibrosing alveolitis :
A. Persistent dry B. Pink frothy
C. Purulent mucoid D. Green viscous

741. On an autopsy specimen of lung tissue, stratified squamous epithelium was noted in the bronchi. Which among the following would best describe its presence
A. Metaplasia B. Hyperplasia
C. Dysplasia D. Hyperplasia

742. Which of the following does not cause interstitial lung disease :
A. Tobacco smoke
B. Sulfur dioxiode
C. Thermophilic actinomycetes
D. Coal dust

Ans.	733. C	734. D	735. D	736. D	737. A	738. A
	739. A	740. A	741. A	742. A	743. C	

743. A patient with history of wheezing, bronchospasm and hemoptysis has bilateral perihilar bronchiectatic shadows on Chest skiagram. The diagnosis is most likely to be :

A. Idiopathic pulmonary fibrosis
B. Sarcoidosis
C. Allergic bronchopulmonary aspergillosis
D. Fibrosing alveolitis

744. The organism most frequently related to the cause of mediastinal fibrosis is :

A. Actinomycosis
B. Histoplasma
C. Hansen bacillus
D. Staphylococcus
E. Koch bacillus

745. Which of the following is not a mediastinal cyst ?

A. Spring water cyst
B. Foregut cyst
C. Pleuropericardial cyst
D. 'Water lily' cyst
E. All of the above

746. Which of the following histological types of lung cancer is associated with the myasthenic (Eaton-Lambert) syndrome?

A. Adenocarcinoma
B. Epidermoid carcinoma
C. Large cell carcinoma
D. Small cell carcinoma

747. Bronchiectasis associated with tuberculosis :

A. Is almost always the direct result of the tuberculous infection
B. In the upper lobes, often represents healed tuberculous cavities
C. Has a different distribution than nontuberculous bronchiectasis
D. Is characterized by the presence of stratified squamous epithelium

748. 'Shock lung' is usually seen :

A. With head injuries
B. With haemorrhagic shock
C. After prolonged cardiopulmonary bypass
D. With multiple trauma
E. All of the above

749. The symptoms of recurrent infection, intractable cough, sputum production, and frequent hemoptysis refractory to medical therapy are indicative of :

A. Oat cell carcinoma of the lung
B. Bronchiectasis
C. Coccidiodomycosis
D. Pulmonary sequestration
E. Empyema

Ans. 744. B 745. D 746. D 647. B 748. E 749. B

750. The most favourable pulmonary metastatic lesions include all except :

A. Breast B. Kidney
C. Testis D. Uterus
E. Melanoma

751. A patient presents with injury to the lower chest, which among the followings is not a correct step in the management :

A. Arrange USS abdomen
B. Intercostal drainage through the second space
C. Caring of # ribs
D. X-ray chest

752. The stage of myasthenia gravis that best responds to thymectomy is :

A. Stage 1 : active B. Stage 2 : inactive
C. Stage 3 : burned out D. Those with thymoma present
E. None of the above

753. Pulmonary neoplasm associated with smoking :

A. Oat cell carcinoma B. Squamous cell carcinoma
C. Adenocarcinoma D. None of the above

754. Aspiration pneumonia most commonly occurs in :

A. Right anterior lobe B. Left postero basal lobe
C. Right upper lobe D. Right lower lobe

755. Surgical intervention in tuberculosis is required for :

A. Hemoptysis B. Miliary tuberculosis
C. Tuberculous empyema D. Tuberculoma

756. Which of the following is the commonest cause of calcified pulmonary metastasis :

A. Adenocarcinoma kidney B. Squamous cell carcinoma
C. Seminoma D. Carcinoma thyroid

757. Which of the following is the commonest tumor of anterior mediastinum :

A. Thymoma B. Neurofibroma
C. Ectopic thyroid D. Lymphoma

758. A case presented with Multisystem trauma with variable blood loss with irregular breathing the diagnosis is :

A. Extradural hematoma B. Rupture lung
C. Spleen rupture D. None of the above

759. A soft tissue tumour causing rib erosion is :

A. Mesothelioma B. Fibrosarcoma
C. Thymoma D. Neurofibroma

Ans.	750. E	751. B	752. A	753. B	754. DDD 755. C
	756. D	75. A	758. B	759. D	

760. Hamman's sign is most characteristic of :
A. Subcutaneous emphysema B. Pneumothorax
C. Pneumopericardium D. Pneumomediastinu

761. Which of the following is true about adenocarcinoma of the bronchus?
A. Is closely associated with pipe smoking
B. Has often spread into the pulmonary veins by the time of diagnosis
C. Equally common in both sexes
D. Account for 25% of bronchogenic carcinomas

762. A patient with aorta-pulmonary fistula characteristically shows all of the following, except :
A. Wide pulse pressure B. Mild cyanosis
C. Cardiomegaly D. Failure to gain weight
E. Frequent respiratory infections

763. The most comon cause of lung abscess is :
A. Failure to use porphylactic antibiotics
B. Chronic atelectasis
C. Aspiration of foreign material
D. Tuberculosis

764. Goals of IPPR are the following except :
A. To maintain PaO2 between 60-80 mm Hg
B. Avoid hypoxia (PaO2 below to 50 mm Hg) or hyperoxia (above PaO2 100 mmHg)
C. Maintain PaCO2 between 35-45 mmHg
D. None of the above

765. Mediastinal bronchogenic cysts are commonest in :
A. Anterior B. Middle
C. Posterior D. Any wher

766. Apnea is defined as cessation of breathing for —— sec or longer or less than —— sec but associated with bradycardia, cyanosis or pallor :
A. 5 B. 10
C. 15 D. 20

767. Cyanosis in which PaO_2 are normal often result due to :
A. Congenital heart disease B. Respiratory disease
C. Valvular lesion D. Abnormal hemoglobin

768. The presence of a post-operative bronchopleural fistula is characterized by all, except :
A. Secondary empyema
B. Pink frothy sputum

Ans.	760. D	781. B	762. B	763. C	764. D	765. A
	766. D	767. D	768. C			

C. Increased coughing in the upright position
D. Symptoms appearing on the 5th or 6th day
E. Spontaneous closure

769. Haemorrhagic pleural effusion with a mass adherent to the chest wall most likely is :
A. Tuberculosis B. Bronchogenic carcinoma
C. Pulmonary infarction D. Mesothelioma
E. Histoplasmosis

770. In a patient of mesothelioma, one often finds :
A. Hypoglycaemia
B. An association with asbestosis
C. Haemorrhagic pleural effusion
D. Clubbing of fingers
E. All of the above

771. Bronchiectasis may develop from all of the following, except :
A. Congenital malformation
B. Chronic pulmonary infection
C. Retained bronchial foreign body
D. Tuberculous
E. Chronic pleural effusion

772. Congenital lobar emphysema is usually treated by :
A. Lobectomy
B. Pneumonectomy
C. Tube drainage
D. Bronchoscopy and aspiration
E. None of the above

773. Thin-walled intra-pulmonary cavities are most frequently associated with :
A. Isoniazid therapy B. Corticosteroid therapy
C. Coccidiodomycosis D. Acute miliary tuberculosis
E. All of the above

774. Pleural fluid with the appearance of anchovy sauce is characteristic of :
A. E. coli B. Entamoeba histolytica
C. Staphylococus aureus D. Echinococcus
E. None of the above

775. The primary treatment of empyema which results from tuberculosis is :
A. Open tube drainage B. Systemic antibiotic therapy
C. Closed tube drainage D. Thoracoplasty
E. Thoracocentesis

Ans.	769. D	770. E	771. E	772. A	773. C	774. B
	775. B					

776. Failure to establish adequate drainage in an empyema with a bronchopleural fistula is indicated by :

A. Drainage less than 100 c.c. per day
B. Haemorrhagic drainage less than 100 c.c per day
C. The development of haemoptysis
D. Continued productive cough with purulent material
E. All of the above

777. Tension Pneumothorax results in :

A. Alkalosis
B. Increased cardiac output
C. Decreased Venous return
D. All of the above

778. The most common fungal disease confused with tuberculosis is :

A. Nacardiosis
B. Coccidiodomycosis
C. Histoplasmosis
D. Actinomycosis
E. Blastomycosis

779. The most common cause of mediastinitis is :

A. Cervical cellulitis
B. Osteomyelitis of vertebrae
C. Pleural empyema
D. Rupture of oesophagus
E. Pericaridits

780. The most frequently causes of haemoptysis :

A. Bronchogenic carcinoma
B. Pulmonary tuberculosis
C. Mitral stenosis
D. Pulmonary embolism
E. Bronchiectasis

781. Most common source for thrombus in Pulmonary Embolism is :

A. Posterior tibial vein
B. Ilio femoral vein
C. Popliteal vein
D. Soleal veins

782. In Pneumothorax due to blunt injury, treatment of choice is :

A. Intercostal drainage
B. Observation
C. Thoractomy
D. Pneumonectomy

783. Chest tubes must not be inserted posterior to :

A. Midaxillary line
B. Posterior axillary line
C. Anterior axillary line
D. Mid-clavicular line

784. Bronchogenic carcinoma commonly metastatise to which endocrine organ :

A. Ovaries
B. Testes
C. Thyroid
D. Adrenals

785. Pleura usually heals in :

A. 1—3 days
B. 3—5 days
C. 5—7 days
D. 21—28 days

786. All of the following are anterior mediastinal tumours except :

A. Thymoma
B. Teratoma
C. Neurofibroma
D. Retrosternal goitre

Ans.	**776. D**	**777. C**	**778. C**	**779. D**	**780. B**	**781. B**
	782. C	**783. B**	**784. D**	**785. C**	**786. C**	

787. A solitary nodule in a chest X-ray is indicative of malignancy if following are present except :

A. The patient is over 45 years

B. Egg shell calcification

C. Indistinct margins
D. Doubing time of 2 weeks

788. Foreign body commonly lodges in :

A. Right lower bronchus
B. Right upper bronchus

C. Left upper bronchus
D. Left lower bronchus

789. Which one of the following is the most important diagnostic physical sign of pneumothorax?

A. Resonant note on percussion with absent or decreased breath sounds

B. Decreased vocal fremitus

C. Making of heart sounds

D. Decreased respiratory movement of chest on the affected side

790. A coin shaped lesion in apical lobes with erosion of ribs and thoracic vertebra is :

A. Coarctation of aorta
B. Pancoast tumour

C. Bronchiectesis
D. Any of the above

791. The following pneumoconiosis has increased risk of developing pleural malignancies :

A. Anthracosis
B. Silicosis

C. Asbestosis
D. Bagassosis

792. All are causes of bilateral common laryngeal nerve palsy except :

A. Thyroid surgery

B. Thyroid malignancy

C. Carcinoma bronchus

D. Carcinoma oesophagus (upper part)

793. Right bronchus is :

A. Short and thin
B. Short and broad

C. Long and broad
D. Long and thin

794. "Frozen chest" usually follows :

A. Emphyema thoracic
B. Pneumothorax

C. Pulmonary tuberculosis
D. Carcinoma transversalis

E. Pleural effusion

795. Injury to recurrent laryngeal nerve produces :

A. Pitch is altered
B. Permanent hoarseness

C. Temporary horseness
D. Stridor

Ans.						
	787. B	788. B	789. A	790. B	791. C	792. D
	793. B	794. A	795. B			

796. Nasogastric suction should be done post-operatively until —— is there :

A. Patient develops sore throat
B. Flatus passed
C. Pulse rate becomes normal
D. No more gastric secretions

797. Post operative atelectasis from obstruction of a major airway may require intrabronchial suction through :

A. Nasotracheal suction B. Direct laryngoscopy
C. Mediastinoscopy D. Endoscopy

798. The mediastinum is shifted to the affected side in

A. Atelectasis B. Pleural effusion
C. Pneumothorax D. Chronic bronchitis

799. Surgery in cases of pulmonary tuberculosis is indicated in all except:

A. Tuberculosis bronchietasis
B. Miliary tuberculosis
C. Tuberculoma of destroyed region
D. Frank destructive lesion not responding to medical treatment

800. The initial treatment of a bacterial lung abscess is :

A. Antibiotic agents, bronchoscopy and postural drainage
B. Lobectomy
C. Open thoracotomy drainage
D. Antibiotic agents followed by resection

801. The ideal way to relieve increasing spontaneous pneumothorax :

A. Suprasternal decompression
B. Thoracotomy
C. Subxiphoid decompression
D. None of the above

802. Which of the following tumours occur commonly in the posterior mediastinum :

A. Thymoma B. Neurofibroma
C. Teratoma D. Pericardial cyst

803. In which of the following ways a patient of chronic empyema of chest can present :

A. Localised empyema
B. Bronchoplerual fistula
C. Discharging sinus at the chest wall
D. All of the above

Ans. **796. B** **797. D** **798. A** **799. B** **800. A** **801. D** **802. B** **803. D**

804. Which one of the following pairs regarding staging of brochogenic carcinoma is not correctly matched

A. Occult carcinoma — TX, NO, MO
B. Stage I — T2, NO, MO
C. Stage II — T3, N1, MO
D. Stage III — T2, N1, M1

805. Regarding development of diaphragm :

A. It develops during 8th week of foetal life
B. Left dome closes later than right
C. It grows partly from pleuroperitoneal fold
D. All the above are true
E. None of the above

806. How long does a part of lung remain unin-flated (atelectatic) in a new born ?

A. Two minutes
B. Two hours
C. Two days
D. Two weeks
E. Two years

807. Which of the following is true regarding Carcinoma bronchus ?

A. Usually presents as haemoptysis
B. Resolves on administration of a course of antibiotics
C. Does not occur in non smokers
D. Should be suspected if a consolidation lungs does not result with all possible treatment for chest infection

808. Which of the following is a contraindication for bronchoscopy ?

A. Emphysema
B. Bronchiectasis
C. Tuberculosis lungs
D. Aortic aneurysm

809. Which of the following is not a contraindication for bronchoscopy ?

A. Lesions of cervical spine
B. Cardiac failure
C. Active bleeding
D. Trismus

810. The most common mediastinal tumour is :

A. Neurogenic tumour
B. Bronchogenic carcinoma
C. Plasma cell myelomas
D. Pericardial cysts

811. Which of the following provides the earliest suggestion of post operative ventillatory failure :

A. Abdominal chest X-ray
B. Rash on the chest wall
C. Restlessness
D. Hyperthermia

812. Which of the following is the most common initial symptom of primary cancer of the hilum of the lung ?

A. Cough
B. Haemoptysis
C. Wheeze
D. Dyspnoea

Ans.					
804. D	805. D	806. D	807. D	808. D	809. C
810. B	811. C	812. A			

813. A 25-year old male is admitted with blunt injury chest. On examination, patient is found to have significant flail chest. The choice of immediate treatment is :

A. Intercostal drainage
B. Tracheal intubation and positive pressure ventilation
C. Aspiration
D. Strapping of chest wall

814. Post operative pulmonary embolism can be pre- vented by all except :

A. Leg exercises
B. Early ambulation
C. Pillows under the calf
D. Compression stockings

815. The sequence of symptoms in pulmonary embolism is :

A. Fever, pain, dyspnoea
B. Fever, dyspnoea, pain
C. Dyspnoea, pain, haemoptysis
D. Dyspnoea, cough, purulent sputum

816. Which one of the following consequences of chest trauma represents the greates immediate threat to life ?

A. Sub-cutaneous emphysema of neck
B. Sucking pneumothorax
C. Tension pneumothorax
D. Haemothorax

817. The commonest cause for not being able to tap out pus in a case of chronic empyema is :

A. Selection of wrong site
B. Use of narrow needle
C. Employment of inefficient syringe
D. Presence of excessive fibrin in pus
E. Clotted pu

818. True position of the intersegmental plane in lungs is indicated by :

A. Pulmonary arteries
B. Pulmonary veins
C. Bronchial arteries
D. None of the above

819. All generations of bronchus are fully present by — week of intrauterine life :

A. 6th
B. 10th
C. 16th
D. 24th

820. Intralobar sequestration of lung is commonest in the :

A. Apical segment of upper lobe
B. Medial segment of middle lobe
C. Lateral basal segment of lower lobe
D. Posterior basal segment of lower lobe

Ans.	**813. B**	**814. C**	**815. C**	**816. B**	**817. A**	**818. A**
	819. C	**820. D**				

821. The diagnosis of haemothorax can be confirmed by :

A. X-ray chest
B. Tomography
C. Thoracoscopy
D. Bronchography
E. None of the above

822. Extralobar bronchogenic cysts may communicate with the following except :

A. Oesophagus
B. Stomach
C. Bronchus
D. None of the above

823. Consider the following statements regarding the involvement of mediastinal lymph nodes in lung cancer :

1. It is detected by CT scan of chest
2. Its enlargement is diagnosed by CT scan of chest
3. Non-homogeneous enhancement of glands is characteristic

Of these statements

A. 1 and 3 are correct
B. 2 and 3 are correct
C. 1 and 2 are correct
D. 1,2 and 3 are correct

824. Commonest cause of spontaenous pneumothorax is :

A. Malignancy
B. Lung abscess
C. Bronchiectasis
D. Rupture of Bulla

825. Most important measure in all serious cases of crush injuries to chest is :

A. Relief of pain
B. Oxygen
C. Tracheostomy
D. Antibiotics

826. The minor degrees of stove-in-chest usually require :

A. Little specific treatment
B. Tracheostomy
C. Surgical correction
D. Positive pressure ventilation

827. The immedaite treatment of choice in most cases of flail chest is :

A. Analgesics
B. Intermittent positive pressure ventillation
C. Tracheostomy
D. Breathing exercises

828. Daily aspirations in mild traumatic haemothorax are usually started after an initial interval of 24 hours as this is the time :

A. When bleeding is not much
B. Blood may not be liquified
C. To allow bleeding vessel to seal
D. None of the above

829. The commonest site of fracture of bronchus is :

A. Upper most part
B. Junction of mediastinal and hilar bronchus
C. Hilar bronchus
D. None of the above

Ans.						
	821. E	822. C	823. A	824. D	825. C	826. A
	827. B	828. C	829. B			

830. "Pump lung" is a term used for :
A. Shock lung resulting due to microthrombo-embolism
B. Shock lung following extensive intravascular coagulation
C. Stiff lung due to markedly decreased lung compliance
D. Shock lung following heart lung bypass

831. Tietz's disease is most common in ——— costal cartilages :
A. 1st, 2nd B. 2nd, 3rd
C. 3rd, 4th D. 4th, 5th

832. The commonest cause of cold abscess of chest wall is :
A. Tuberculous intercostal lymphadenitis
B. Pott's spine
C. TB of ribs
D. TB of sternum

833. Cold abscess is chest most commonly presents in the :
A. Anterior axillary line B. Midaxillary line
C. Posterior axillary line D. Spine

834. For pleurodesis, the following may be used except :
A. Silver nitrate (5%) B. Iodised talc
C. Comphor in oil (0.5%) D. Ethyl alcohol (20%)

835. Fluid in pleural effusion first collects at : AIIMS 1984
A. Anterir costophrenic angle
B. Posterior costophrenic angle
C. Parasternal area
D. Any of the above

836. Normal amount of pleural fluid is approximately :
A. 5 ml B. 15 ml
C. 50 ml D. 100 ml

837. A majority of surgically produced chylous effusions require the following measures except :
A. Low fat diet
B. Chest aspiration
C. Thoracotomy and suturing
D. None of the above

838. The following may arise anywhere in the mediasti-num except :
A. Tuberculous adenitis B. Secondaries
C. Sarcoids D. Teratoma

839. Which is the commonest congenital anomaly of diaphragm :
A. Eventration
B. Oesophageal hiatus hernia
C. Hernia through forament of Morgagni
D. Hernia through foramen of Bochdalek

Ans.	830. D	831. B	832. A	833. A	834. D	835. B
	836. A	837. C	838. D	839. B		

840. Biot's respiration is seen in :

A. Hypnosedative poisoning B. Appendicitis

C. Cholecystitis D. Bulbar poliomyelitis

841. The one which does not require cardiopulmonary bypass is :

A. M S with M R B. VSD

C. Fallot's tetrology D. PDA

842. All of the following may produce the thoracic outlet syndrome except :

A. Cervical rib B. Costoclavicular compression

C. Raynaud's disease D. Scalenus anticus syndrome

843. Closed tracheal injury due to trauma most often involves the trachea or bronchi near the :

A. Cricoid B. Mid-trachea

C. Carina D. Secondary bronchi

844. A 20-year-old man falls from the roof of a two- storey building, landing on a heap of rubble. The initial evaluation reveals a flail chest to be the only obvious injury. The patient is in severe respiratory distress with tachypnoea (rate = 40/minute). The percussion note is bilaterally symmetrical and the breath sounds on the right side are slightly decreased. Arterial blood gases on facemask oxygen are : PaOz, 45 mmHg; PaCo2 mmHg and pH 7.47. Which component of his injury is most likely to have caused these abnormal blood gases ?

A. Chest wall instability B. Hypovolaemia

C. Pain D. Pulmonary contusion

845. Fluoroscopically guided transthoracic needle biopsy of lung is least useful in :

A. Central lesiòns less than 2 cm in size

B. Peripheral lesions less than 1 cm

C. Cavitating lesions in all position

D. All of the above are equal

846. The incidence of neoplastic degeneratịon is greater in :

A. Infant pulmonary hamatomas

B. Adult pulmonary hamartomas

C. Both of the above all equal

D. Neither of the above malignant tendencies

847. Amoebic lung abscess is commonly due to :

A. Direct extension B. Haematogenous spread

C. Lymphatic spread D. From liver

Ans.	840. B	841. D	842. C	843. C	844. A	845. A
	846. D	847. A				

848. Post operative pneumonia is most commonly due to :
A. Gram negative bacilli B. Streptococcus
C. Staphyloccoccus D. Mycoplasma

849. Ca lung mainly metastasize to :
A. Liver B. Brain
C. Bone D. Skin

850. Lung carcinoma and nonsmoking indicates :
A. Multifactorial etiology B. Unifactorial etiology
C. Unpredictable associatio D. No association

851. Pancoast tumor produces :
A. Marked Erythema B. Horner's syndrome
C. Monoplegia D. Hemiparesis

852. The most common type of bronchogenic carcinoma is :
A. Epidermoid B. Anaplastic
C. Alveolar D. Bronchiolar

853. Contraindications to PEEP include all except :
A. Pulmonary oedema B. Emphysema
C. Cardiogenic shock D. Pneumoni

854. Treatment of flail chest include all, except :
A. Tracheostomy to reduce dead space
B. Positive pressure respiration
C. Traction on the broken fragments of ribs
D. Internal fixation of fragments by wire

855. Treatment of 10% spontaneous pneumo-thorax is :
A. Observation B. Immediate thoracotomy
C. Tube thoracostomy D. Endotracheal intubation

856. Prolonged postoperative respiratory support is better provided by :
A. Volume cycled respirators
B. Pressure cycled respirators
C. Both of the above are equal
D. Neither of the above

857. Paradoxical respiration is seen in :
A. Flail chest B. Tension pneumothorax
C. Empyema necessitans D. Mediastinal emphysema

858. Dyspnea, chest pain, hypoglycemia, hypertrophic pulmonary osteoarthropathy and a hemorrhagic pleural effusion is most likely in :
A. Pulmonary tuberculosis B. Alveolar cell carcinoma
C. Metatatic thymoma D. Mesothelioma

Ans.	848. A	849. A	850. A	851. B	852. A	853. A
	854. C	855. A	856. A	857. A	858. D	

859. All are true with bronchial adenoma except :
A. Uncommon benign tumours of the bronchus
B. 10% of them are malignant
C. 80% of them arise from a major bronchus
D. They produce localized emphysema

860. Empyema necessitans is defined as a pleural em-pyema which :
A. Is under pressure
B. Has ruptured into the bronchus
C. Has ruptured into the pericardium
D. Is showing extension to the subcutaneous tissue

861. The greatest incidence of bronchopleural fistula is following :
A. Segmental resection B. Lobectomies
C. Pneumonectomies D. Thoracotomy

862. The most useful investigation in the diagnosis of bronchiectasis is :
A. Pulmonary angiography B. Bronchography
C. Arterial blood gases D. Lungs can

863. Brochiogenic lung cysts are due to :
A. Metastatic carcinoma
B. Klebsella infection
C. Abnormal budding of the bronchial buds
D. Chest trauma

864. Horner's syndrome assocaited with pain shoulder and arm is suggestive of :
A. Aortic aneurysm B. Myocardial infarction
C. Cervical Spondylosis D. Pancoast's tumour
E. Shoulder girdle syndrome

865. Common cause of microabscesses in lungs inclues :
A. Streptococcus B. Staphylococcus
C. Pneumococcus D. Klebsiella

866. Hoarseness of voice when present alongwith a suspected abnormal mediastinal mass shadow is probably due to :
A. Mediastinal lymphadenitis
B. An abscess in midiastinum
C. Aortic aneurysm
D. Carcinoma oesophagus

867. Which of the following often metastasizes to opposte lung?
A. Epidermoid carcinoma B. Alveolar cell carcinoma
C. Adenocarcinoma D. Carcinoid

868. Muscle not cut in posterolateral thoracotomy is :
A. Serratus ant. B. Latissimus dorsi
C. Rhomboides major D. Serratus posterior sup.

Ans.						
	859. A	**860. D**	**861. C**	**862. D**	**863. C**	**864. D**
	865. B	**866. C**	**867. C**	**868. C**		

869. Chest tubes must not be inserted posterior to :
A. Mid-axillary line B. Posterior axillary line
C. Anterior axillary line D. Mid clavicular line

870. Intrabronchial foreign bodies may require which of the following :
A. Bronchoscopy B. Bronchotomy
C. Lung resection D. All of the above

871. The Chemotherapy is most useful for :
A. Squamous cell carcinoma B. Oat cell carcinoma
C. Adenocarcinoma D. Neuroblastoma

872. Best treatment for thoracic duct rupture is :
A. Operative correction B. Fat emulsion
C. Observation D. Antibiotics

873. Thoracotomy is best indicated in :
A. Cardiac temponade
B. Multiple fracture of ribs
C. Multiple fracture of ribs with hemothorax
D. Spontaneous pneumothorax

874. Which of the following primaries do not produce a smooth secondary in lungs :
A. Seminoma B. Carcinoma lymph node
C. Carcinoma thyroid D. Carcinoma lung

875. Multiple interstitial nodules are not seen in :
A. Miliary tuberculosis B. Tropical eosinophilia
C. Lobar pneumonia D. Asbestosis

876. Three most common symptoms of bronchogenic carcinoma are the following except :
A. Cough with sputum for more than 2-3 weeks
B. Pain chest
C. Haemoptysis
D. Dyspnoea

877. Adson's manuovre is employed to detect :
A. Thoracic outlet obstruction
B. Incompetent saphenofemoral junction
C. Site of AV malformation
D. Deep vein thrombus site

878. Commonest cause of hydropneumothorax in our country is :
A. Broncheogenic carcinoma
B. Sarcoidosis
C. Emphysematous bulla
D. Pulmonary tuberculosis

Ans.	869. B	870. D	871. B	872. C	873. C	874. B
	875. C	876. B	877. A	878. C		

879. Commonest indication for surgery in pectus excavatum is :
A. Recurrent respiratory infections
B. Respiratory deficiency
C. Cosmetic reasons
D. Presses great vessels

880. Treatment of choice in severe flail chest is :
A. Inter costal block
B. Strapping + analgesics
C. Fixation of fractured ribs with wire
D. Intermittent positive pressure ventilation

881. An infant achieves adult levels of Pulmonary vascular resistance and pulmonary artery pressure by age :
A. Birth B. 1-3
C. 3-6 D. 6-12

882. The cause of massive haemoptysis is :
A. Tuberculosis B. Viral pneumonia
C. Bronchiectesis D. Bronchogenic carcinoma

883. Cavity formation in bronchogenic carcinoma occurs in :
A. Oat cell carcinoma B. Squamous cell carinoma
C. Adenocarcinoma D. Bronchoalveolar carcinoma

884. Open drainage of empyema is indicated only :
A. In streptococcal infections
B. When the pus is thick
C. When the mdiastinum is fixed
D. In bilateral disease
E. When thoracostomy tube drainage is ineffective

885. In an unconsicious patient following multiple injuries resulting due to an accident after taking alcohol, the following is preferred :
A. Endotracheal tube (uncuffed)
B. Endotrocheal tube (cuffed)
C. Tracheostomy
D. Oropharyngeal tube

886. Blood stained sputum may be the only symptom in :
A. Bronchiectasis B. Carcinoma bronchus
C. Adenoma bronchus D. Pulmonary TB

887. Investigation of choice in pulmonary embolism is :
A. Chest X-ray B. Ultrasound
C. CT Scan D. Ventilation-perfusion scan

888. Bronchogenic carcinoma which produce paraneo-plastic syndrome :
A. Squamous cell carcinoma B. Oat cell carcinoma
C. Adenocarcinoma D. Large cell carcinoma

Ans.	879. C	880. D	881. D	882. C	883. B	884. C
	885. B	886. C	887. D	888. B		

889. Treatment of recurrent pulmonary embolism in adults includes all except :

A. Mobin Udin umbrella
B. Kimray Greenfield filter
C. Plication of IVC
D. Femoral thromboembolectomy

890. Treatment of uncomplicated hydatid cyst in lung is :

A. Marsupialisation B. Lobectomy
C. Enucleation D. Extended tube drainage

891. Spontaneous rupture of a major bronchus would cause all except :

A. Massive pneumothorax B. Haemothorax
C. Subcutaenous emphysem D. Mediastinal emphysema

892. In patient suspected to have suffered a pulmonary embolism, immediate primary treatment consists of :

A. Pulmonary embolectomy
B. Infusion of streptokinase
C. Anticoagulant drugs
D. Inferior vena caval clipping

893. The clinical features of thoracic outlet syndrome include all of the following except :

A. Paresthesia along the ulnar border
B. Ischaemic gangrene of the digits
C. Atrophy and wasting of the thenar eminence
D. Bruit in the neck

894. Following an operation a pt. developed pulmonary rupture. Sign is :

A. Dyspnoeic with slow pulseB. Tachycardia
C. Haemoptysis D. Asymptomatic

895. Most common cause of acute mediastinitis is :

A. Oesophageal rupture
B. Tracheal rupture
C. Inflammation of thoracic vertebra
D. Fracture of ribs

896. Quantitative estimation of Air embolism is by :

A. Doppler B. Pulmonary wedge pressure
C. End tidal CO2 estimation D. ECG

897. Young male with accident - massive left sided haemothorax. Immediate treatment is :

A. Tube thoracostomy
B. Strapping
C. Endotracheal intubation, IPPV and pleural aspiration
D. Observation

Ans.	889. C	890. C	891. B	892. B	893. C	894. A
	895. C	896. B	897. C			

898. **All of the following are cavitating lesions of lung except :**
A. Sq. cell carcinoma
B. Caplan's syndrome
C. Hamartoma
D. Wegner's granulomatosis

899. **Least likely cause of lung secondaries is :**
A. Ca breast
B. Ca testis
C. Ca ovary
D. Ca prostate

900. **Which is true regarding adenocaricnoma of lung :**
A. Cause 50% of lung cancers
B. More common in females
C. Associated with subcutaneous angio-myolipomas
D. Peripheral location

901. **Majority of lung cysts cccur :**
A. Near the carina
B. In Mediastinum
C. Peribronchial tissue
D. Base

902. **Most common sign of aspiration pneumonitis :**
A. Tachypnoea
B. Bronchospasm
C. Cyanosis
D. Crepitations

903. **Intralobar sequestration of lung gets its blood supply from :**
A. Descending aorta
B. Pulmonary artery
C. Internal mammary artery
D. None of the above

904. **B/L diphragmatic paralysis which is not true :**
A. Causes normocapnic failure
B. Shift test is positive in fluoroscopy
C. Diaphgramic pacing may be helpful
D. None of the above

905. **Commonest complication of blunt injury thorax :**
A. Aortic rupture
B. Pneumothorax
C. Haemopneumothorax
D. # rib

906. **Rx of choice of post operative lung collapse :**
A. Endoscopic suction
B. Pulmonary resection
C. Corticosteroids
D. Needle drainage

907. **A young female patient has been admitted following a road accident with complaints of pain in the right side of the chest. On examination she is found to have rapid and shallow breathing, a fast pulse rate and hyper-rosonant chest with absent breath sound on the right side. The most appropriate immediate course of action would be to :**
A. Perform a diagnostic chest aspiration on right side and put in a chest tube
B. Order for urgent chest X-ray and start oxygen
C. Put the patient on positive pressure ventilation
D. Send for the cardiothoracic surgeon for exploraton of chest

Ans.	898. B	899. D	900. D	901. A	902. A	903. A
	904. A	905. D	906. A	907. A		

908. Eventration of diaphragm does not occur in :

A. Vagotomy
B. Post-lobectomy
C. Phrenic nerve palsy
D. Mediastinal mass

909. Commonest symptom associated with thoracic outlet syndrome is :

A. Intermittent claudication
B. Pain in radial nerve distribution
C. Pain in ulnar nerve distribution
D. Gangrene

910. The following are the indications for the tube thoracostomy of parapneumonic effusion, except :

A. Pleural fluid glucose evel less than 50mg/dl
B. Presence of gross amount of pus in the plural space
C. Organism visible on gram stain of pleural fluid
D. Pleural fluid pro is more than 3gm/dl

911. A patient aspirated a foreign body in the standing position. Where is it likely to lodge :

A. Right anterobasal
B. Right medial basal
C. Right posterobasal
D. Right lateral basal

912. Commonest cause of Hypotension in fracture ribs (T10-T12) :

A. Intercostal artery damage
B. Pulmonary confusion
C. Abdominal solid visceral organ injury
D. Damage to aorta

913. In hiatus hernia with haematemesis, the cause is likely to be :

A. Reflux esophagitis
B. Chr. duodenal ulcer
C. Variceal blood
D. Chr. gastritis

914. The commonest tumor associated with acquired pure red cell aplasia is :

A. Bronchogenic carcinoma
B. Hepatic carcinoma
C. Hodgkin's lymphoma
D. Thymoma

915. A patient presents with respiratory distress, hypotension and dilated bulging neck veins after chest trauma, most likely cause is :

A. Hemothorax
B. Tension Pneumothorax
C. Flail chest
D. None of the above

916. All of the following regarding Bochdalech hernia is true except :

A. Early respiratory distress leading to early diagnosis and treatment are good prognostic sign
B. Common on left posterior side
C. Stomach and transverse colon are commonest content to herniate
D. Diagnosed prenatally by ultrasound

Ans.	908. D	909. C	910. D	911. A	912. A	913. A
	914. D	915. B	916. A			

917. **A patient having fever, heaviness in chest and difficulty in breathing was found to have pleural effusion, chest drain has to be put in .Most common site of drainage is :**
   A. 2nd intercostal space midclavicular line
   B. 5th intercostal space just lateral to vertebral column
   C. 7th intercostal midaxillary line
   D. 5th intecostal space midclavicular line

918. **After thyroid surgery, patient developed sudden respiratory distress, dressing was removed and it was found to be slightly blood stained and wound was bulging. First thing to do is :**
   A. Remove the stitch and take the patient to O.T.
   B. Laryngoscopy and intubation
   C. Tracheostomy
   D. Cricothyroidotomy

919. **Which of the following features denote a contraindication for surgical resection in a case of carcinoma lung :**
   A. Malignant pleural effusion
   B. Involvement of visceral pleura
   C. Hilar lymphadenopathy
   D. Consolidation of one lobe

920. **Lalloo, a 55 year old chronic smoker, presents with complaints of hoarseness of voice. On examination there is a single enlarged painless lymphnode in the left supraclavicular area. What is the next step to be done :**
   A. Excision biopsy of the node
   B. Laryngoscopy and chest X-ray
   C. CT scan of chest
   D. Sputum for AFB

921. **True statement about thoracic outlet syndrome is :**
   A. Results from compression of brachial artery and brachial plexus
   B. Neurological symptoms are seen in distributionof C5 and sC6
   C. Occurs due to compression of neurovascular bundle between insertion of anterior and middle scalenus muscle
   D. None of the above

922. **60 year old man with suspected bronchogenic Ca: TB has been ruled out in this patient. What investigation would be chosen :**
   A. CT guided FNAC
   B. Bronchoscopy and biopsy
   C. X-ray
   D. Sputum examination

923. **Clotted haemothorax is treated by :**
   A. Rib resection
   B. Tube drainage
   C. Injection of streptokinase
   D. Surgery

Ans. 917. C 918. A 919. A 920. B 921. C 922. B 923. D

924. Consider the following statements :

1. Pharyngeal diverticulum is aprotrusion of pouch through the neck defect called Killian's sehiscence
2. It is initiated by imperfect relaxation of strap muscles
3 It is common in mated & usually presents as a left sided neck swelling
4. Cricopharyngeal myotomy is an essential compovent of its surgical procedure

Which of these statements are correct for pharyngeal diverticulum :

A. 1, 2 & 4 B. 1, 3 & 4
C. 1, 2 & 3 D. 3 & 4

925. The following are true about bronchogenic carcinoma except :

A. It is the commonest malignant tumour in men
B. One-Lung-Anaesthesia has improved results of surgery
C. Most lung cancers are unresectable at presentation
D. Small cell carcinoma carries better survival rate

926. A post operative cardiac surgical patient developed sudden hypotension, raised central venous pressure, pulsus paradoxus at the 4th post-operative hour. The most probabale diagnosis is :

A. Excessive mediastinal bleeding
B. Ventricular dysfunction
C. Congestive cardiac failure
D. Cardiac tamonade

927. 'Popcorn' calcification in a lung nodule is pathognomic of :

A. Hamartomas B. Histoplasmosis
C. Tuberculosis D. Benign nodule

928. A 60 year old male was diagnosed as carcinoma right lung. On CECT chest there was a tumor of 5´5 cm in upper lobe and another 2´2 cms size tumor nodule in middle lobe. The primary modality of treatment is?

A. Radiotherapy B. Chemotherapy
C. Surgery D. Supportive treatment

929. In which of the following conditions is Paradoxical respiration observed ?

A. Stove- in - chest B. Flail chest
C. Pneumothorax D. Haemopneumothorax

930. Poorest prognosis in lung cancer is associated with :

A. Small cell carcinoma
B. Squamous cell carcinoma
C. Squamous cell carcinoma
D. Adenosquamous carcinoma

Ans.	924. B	925. D	926. D	927. A	928. C	929. B
	930. A					

931. An elevated right hemidiaphram following abdomi-nal trauma should suggest:

A. Rupture of liver
B. Rupture of diaphgram
C. Right lower lobe atelectassis
D. Subpleural fluid

932. On serial chest film a nodule with tumour doubling time of over one year increase the probability that the lesion is :

A. Cystic
B. Malignant
C. Benign
D. Inflammatory

933. Dilatation of upper lobe vein is a reliable sign of :

A. Hilar Tumour
B. Emphysema
C. Pulmonary hypertention
D. Cardiac decompensation.

934. Chylothorax is associated with all except :

A. Whipple's disease
B. Hodgkin's disease
C. Pulmonary lymphangiomyomatosis
D. Blunt chest trauma
E. Lymphangitis carcinomatosis

935. Water lilly appearance in chest X-ray is suggestive of :

A. Bronchiectasis
B. Bronchopleural fistula
C. Hydatid cyst
D. Sequestration cyst of lung

936. In a child, pneumatocoele formation is seen in all except:

A. Escherichia coli pneumonia
B. Streptococcal pneumonia
C. Hydrocarbon ingestion
D. Goodpasture's syndrome
E. Tuberculosis

937. Hypertrophic pulmonary osteoarthropathy occurs with following except:

A. Fibrosing alveolitis
B. Pleural fibroma
C. Squamous carcinoma of the bronchus
D. Myeloma depositis in ribs

938. Increased radiolucency of one sided hemithorax may be caused by following except :

A. Expiratory films
B. Pneumothorax
C. Patient rotatio
D. Obstructive emphysema.

939. Normal pulmonary arterial pressure (mmHg) in systole is :

A. 10 - 12
B. 12 - 16
C. 16 - 20
D. 25 - 30
E. 30 - 35

Ans. **931. B** **932. C** **933. D** **934. A** **935. C** **936. D**
937. D **938. A** **939. D**

940. Calcification in pulmonary metastases may be found most often in:

A. Osteosarcoma
B. Papillary carcinoma thyroid
C. Chondrosarcoma
D. Ovarian cystadenoma
E. Carcinoma of breast.

941. Local tracheal displacement in the neck is most commonly due to :

A. Marked Pleural effusion B. Atelectesis
C. Enlarged thyroid D. Thyroiditis
E. Cyst.

942. The most common underlying scar for scar carcinoma in lungs is:

A. Infaract B. Granuloma
C. Tuberculoma D. Fibrotic scar.

943. Typical carcinoid in lung presents as :

A. Lobar collapse B. Obstructive pneumonitis
C. Hilar mass D. Any of the above.

944. Pneumothorax is not a feature in:

A. Honeycomb lungs B. Bronchietasis
C. Tuberculosis D. Emphysema

945. Round pneumonias occur in :

A. Children B. Adult males
C. Adult females D. Elderly

946. Cavitating pulmonary metastases are usually from:

A. Testes B. Colon
C. Kidneys D. Cervix

947. The following are the cardiophrenic angle masses except:

A. Pericardial cyst
B. Diaphgramatic hernia through formamen of Morgagni
C. Epicardial nodes
D. Bronchogenic cyst.

948. Fibrosing mediastinitis may result due to:

A. Tuberculosis B. Histoplasmosis
C. Iatrogenic D. Any of the above.

949. Primary lung cancer is unlikely if a solitary pulmonary nodule:

A. Has well-defined margins
B. Has spiculated margins
C. Contains pleural tag
D. There is no growth for at least 2 years.

Ans.	940. A	941. C	942. A	943. D	944. A	945. A
	946. D	947. D	948. D	949. D		

950. Pancoast tumour is more commonly seen in type:
A. Squamous B. Columnar
C. Adeno D. Pseudostratified

951. The intensity of colour in Doppler is determined by :
A. Direction of flow
B. Velocity of flow
C. Strength of returning echo
D. Duration of flow

952. Kerley's A& B lines are:
A. Thickened interlobular septa
B. Linear atelectatic lung shadow
C. Vascular shadow
D. Lymphatic shadow.

953. Pulmonary embolism is best diagnosed by :
A. CT Scan B. Ventilation -perfusion scan
C. X-ray Chest D. Pulmonary function

954. Following truama to the chest, an increasing hemothorax suggest that bleeding source:
A. From pulmonary vessel. B. Unrelated to truama
C. From the lung D. Not from the lung.

955. The best view of the chest to show minimal sub pulmonary effusion is :
A. PA view B. AP view
C. Lateral decubitus view D. Oblique view

956. Middle lobe collapse may be demonstrateded to best advantage on the :
A. Frontal projection B. Lateral projection
C. Lordotic projection D. Overexposed view.

957. A pulmonary consolidation in a patient with asthma is frequently due to :
A. Aspergillosis B. Fibrosis
C. Tuberculosis D. Cryptococcosis

958. One of primary differential points between pulmonary embolism and infarction is :
A. Clear lung fields B. Diaphragmatic change
C. Pleural fluid D. Hilar change

959. Persistent bilateral pulmonary change associated with acute renal failure accure in except:
A. Churge-Strauss syndrome B. Goodpasture's syndrome
C. Wegener's granulomatosis D. Acute pyelonephritis
E. Systemic lupus erythematosis

Ans.	950. A	951. C	952. A	953. B	954. D	955. C
	956. C	957. A	958. A	959. D		

960. **Pneumothorax is best demonstrated by taking a radiograph, with the patient in:**
A. Inspiration
B. Expiration
C. Full inspiration
D. Full expiration
E. Supine.

961. **During angiocardiography, accidental injection of contrast into the myocardium is :**
A. Usually fatal
B. Markedly well tolerated
C. A common caues of ventricular fibrillation
D. Always followed by severe myocardial damage

962. **The cause of single coin shadow in the lung with calcification in the center is :**
A. Epidermoid carcinoma
B. Adeno carcinoma
C. Melanoma
D. Oat cell tumour

963. **Oligaemic lung fields are seen in all of the following except:**
A. Tetralogy of Fallot
B. Anomalous venus drainage
C. Tricuspid stenosis
D. Atrial septal defects.

964. **Sign of greatest value in diagnosis of pulmonary emphysema is :**
A. Hyperlucency
B. Hyperaeration
C. Change in calibre of arteries
D. Diaphragm depression

965. **Most direct and reliable roentgen sign of lobar collapse is :**
A. Air bronchogram
B. Displacement of interlobar septum
C. Mediastinal shift
D. Radio density.

966. **Primary importance of air bronchogram is to localise intrathoracic lesion as being :**
A. Pneumonitis
B. Atelectasis
C. Intrapulmonary
D. Extrapulmonary

967. **The lordotic view is valuable in confirming the presence of lesion in the lung apex and also in the :**
A. Posterior mediastinum
B. Lingular segment
C. Posterior basal segment
D. Hilum

Ans.	960. D	961. B	962. A	963. D	964. C	965. B
	966. C	967. B				

968. The expiratory film is valuable in detecting a small pneumothorax because:

A. Pleural pressure is fixed
B. Pleural pressure is diminished
C. Intra pulmonary pressure is diminished
D. Intrapulmonary pressure is increased.

969. Childhood tuberculosis is most often characterized by:

A. Pleural effusion
B. Infiltrate and nodal enlargment.
C. Hilar enlargment and pleural fluid
D. Cavity lesions and hilar adenopathy.

970. Bilateral calcification in lungs can occur in all except:

A. Friedlanders pneumonia
B. Coccidiodomycosis
C. Histoplasmosis
D. Pulmonary tuberculosis.

971. Causes of a cavitating lesion in the chest radiograph are except:

A. Harmartoma
B. Pulmonary infarction
C. Squamous carcinoma of the bronchus
D. Capaln's syndrome
E. Haematoma

972. Most frequent finding following a fracture of the trachea or bronchus is :

A. Pneumothorax
B. Interstitial air
C. Deviation of trachea
D. Pleural fluid

973. The nodular pattern often seen in the lungs following renal transplantation is thought to be due to :

A. Fungus
B. Infarcts
C. Cytomegalovirus
D. Autoimmune reaction.

974. Most reliable sign of diaphragmatic paralysis:

A. Positive sniff test
B. Unequal movement
C. Elevated diaphgram
D. Mediastinal shift

975. Pneumography is a method of examination for peritoneal or retroperitoneal structure; gas used as contrast agent in this examination is :

A. Oxygen
B. Nitrogen
C. Carbon dioxide
D. Any of the above.

976. Origin of Pulmonary metastasis is maximum from :

A. Kidney
B. Head and Neck
C. Ovary
D. Breast

Ans.	968. C	969. B	970. A	971. A	972. B	973. C
	974. D	975. C	976. D			

977. Ossific nodules in the lungs have been observed in:

A. Constructive pericarditis B. Left artial myxoma

C. Mitral stenosis D. All of the above.

978. Calcification can occur in pulmonary metastases from the following except in :

A. Carcinoma of the pancreas

B. Carcinoma of the breast

C. Adenocarcinoma of the thyroid

D. Squamous cell carcinoma

E. Papillary cystadenomcarcinom of the ovary.

979. Progressive massive fibrosis can occur in:

A. Bagassosis B. Beryllosis

C. Soilicosis D. Stannosis

980. Fluoroscopy is indicated in the following:

A. Chronic pulmonary tuberculosis.

B. Early pulmonary tuberculosis

C. Acute miliary tuberculosis

D. In patient with specific complaints referable to chest.

981. The most common cause of spontaneous pneumo-thorax is:

A. Tuberculosis

B. Bronchial adenoma

C. Bronchogenic carcinoma

D. Rupture of a subpleural bleb.

982. The following may result in miliary shadows on chest X-ray except:

A. Sarcoidosis

B. Mitral Stenosis

C. Pnemoconoisis

D. Staphylococcal pneumonia.

983. The most common malignant tumour of the lung in smokers is:

A. Fibrosarcoma B. Adenocarcinoma

C. Leiomyosarcoma D. Squamous cell carcinoma.

984. Smoking causes ———— emphyrema :

A. Panacinar B. Centriacinar

C. Irregular D. Rare septal

985. One of the following causes mediastinal enlargement:

A. Diffused histiocytic lymphoma

B. Lymphoblastic lymphoma

C. Premyelocytic leukemia

D. CLL

Ans.	977. D	978. D	979. C	980. D	981. D	982. B
	983. D	984. B	985. A			

986. Cavitating lung lesions are seen in following except :

A. Osteosarcoma
B. Histoplasma
C. Silicosis
D. Sarcoidosis

987. Opaque hemithorax is seen in:

A. Emphysema thoracis
B. Bronchopneumonia
C. Aspiration of Foreign body
D. Hypoplasia lungs

988. The Number of bronchopulmonry segments in man :

A. 12 on Rt side, 11 on Lt side
B. 12 on Rt side, 10 on Lt side
C. 10 of each side
D. 10 on Rt side, 8 on Lt side

989. Pneumomediastinum can be seen in all except :

A. Legionnaires disease
B. Ketoacidosis
C. Histiocytosis
D. Duodenal perforation
E. Respiratory distress syndrome.

990. The most common type of carcinoma lung in females and non-smokers is:

A. Squamous cell carcinoma
B. Adenocarcinoma
C. Small cell
D. Large cell

991. The following diseases generally affect the lower zones except:

A. Asbestosis
B. Eosinophilic granuloma
C. Scleroderma
D. Rheumatoid arthritis.

992. The following are interstitial disease of large lung volumes except:

A. Cystic fibrosis
B. Eosinophoilic granuloma
C. Lymphangiomyomatosis
D. None of the above

993. The differential diagnosis of Honey comb lung include the following :

A. Eosinophilic granuloma
B. Sarcoidosis
C. Pneumonconiosis
D. All of the above

994. Bronchorrhea is characteristically seen in :

A. Sarcoidosis
B. Scleroderma
C. Bronchoalveolar carcinoma
D. Goodpasture's syndrome

995. Alveolar proteinosis commonly lead to :

A. Honeycomb lung
B. Interstitial disease of large lung volume
C. Diffuse air-space disease
D. All of the above

Ans.						
	986. D	**987. D**	**988. D**	**989. A**	**990. B**	**991. B**
	992. D	**993. D**	**994. C**	**995. C**		

996. In adults, the commonest lesion in thoracic inlet is :

A. Substernal thyroid B. Teratoma
C. Thymoma D. Lymphoma

997. Malignant thymoma most commonly spreads to :

A. Brain B. Spine
C. Pleura D. Liver

998. About -------- % of patients with thymoma have myasthenia gravis and ---------- % of patients with myaesthenia gravis have thymo mas :

A. 15,25 B. 25,15
C. 50,15 D. 90,50

999. "Golden S" Sign is seen in :

A. Right upper lobe collapse
B. Left upper lobe collapse
C. Right middle lobe collapse
D. Lower lob collapse

1000. Maximal coronal diameters of trachea in males and females are ------ mm respectively :

A. 25, 23 B. 27, 25
C. 25, 21 D. 23, 20

1001. Translucent hemithorax on chest X-ray is seen in:

A. Senile emphysema
B. Fallot's tetralogy
C. Pulmonary hypertension
D. Poliomyelitis

1002. Recurrent pneumothoraces is associated with the following except :

A. Scleroderma B. Histyocystosis X
C. Apical pleural bulla D. Endometriosis
E. None of the above.

1003. All are superior mediastinal tumors except:

A. Thymoma
B. Pleurodermoid cyst
C. Branchial cyst
D. Extra-adrenal phaeochromocytoma

1004. Anterior displacement of the trachea may be due to all of the following except:

A. Mediastinitis B. Achlasia Cardia
C. Zenker's diverticulum D. Neuroenteric Cyst
E. Aneurysm of ascending aorta.

Ans.	996. A	997. C	998. C	999. A	1000. B	1001. D
	1002. E	1003. C	1004. E			

1005. In pulmonary sarcoidosis, the most prodominant finding in X-ray chest is involvement of :

A. Right paratracheal lymph nodes
B. Lungs in a symmetrical fashion
C. Lungs in asymmetrical fashion
D. Mediastinal Nodes
E. Lung parenchyma and mediastinal nodes.

1006. Perihilar fluffy opacities on chest X-ray are seen in :

A. Pulmenary venous hypertention
B. Pulmonary arterial hypertension
C. Pulmonary embolism
D. Pericardial effusion

1007. Best position for chest X-ray to detect left pleural effusion is :

A. Right lateral decubitus B. Left lateral decubitus
C. Left lateral D. Supine

1008. In Emphysema, chest X-ray shows :

A. Nodular opacity
B. Increased bronchovascular markings
C. Multiple cystic airways
D. Wide intercostal spaces

1009. Kerley-B-Lines are seen when pulmonary venous pressure is :

A. 8 mm Hg B. 20 mm Hg
C. 25 mm Hg D. 40 mm Hg

1010. The investigation of choice for minimum pericardial effusion is :

A. Lat. decubitus X-ray B. Ultrasound
C. Echocardiography D. ECG

1011. Air bronchogram is seen in:

A. Lung abscess B. Lung cavity
C. Pneumothorax D. Consolidation

1012. Middle lobe postural drainage is done in which position:

A. Lateral decubitus
B. Supine
C. Prone
D. Sitting and bending forward

1013. `Apical cap sign' is seen in :

A. Supravalvular AS B. PDA
C. Mesothelioma D. Extrapleural haematoma

1014. Right lung is seen best in the following view:

A. Right posterior oblique B. Right anterior oblique
C. Left anterior oblique D. Lateral

Ans.	1005. B	1006. A	1007. B	1008. D	1009. C	1010. C
	1011. D	1012. A	1013. D	1014. B		

1015. Pleural effusion without evident lung infiltration is most often due to :

A. Viral pleurisy B. Carcinoma
C. Lymphom D. Tuberculosis

1016. Tracheal bifurcation is best visualised on which standard view of the chest:

A. Left anterior oblique B. Left posterior oblique
C. Right anterior oblique D. Right post. oblique

1017. Inversion of left hemidiaphragm and paradoxical movement may be due to :

A. Pleural fibrosis B. Cardiomegaly
C. Diaphragmatic paralysis D. Pleural fluid

1018. X-ray of ant. mediastinum does not show :

A. Teratoma B. Neurofibroma
C. Thymic tumors D. Pleuropericardial cyst

1019. Patchy consolidation with hilar lymphadenitis in a child is due to :

A. Tuberculosis B. Whooping cough
C. Measles D. All of the above

1020. Most common cause for pneumothorax :

A. Penetrating trauma
B. Mechanical ventilation
C. Diffuse pulmonary disease
D. Spontaneous

1021. Pleural calcification is seen in :

A. Asbestosis B. Bronchiectesis
C. MS D. Pulm. eosinophilia

1022. Modified lateral decubitus radiograph of chest can detect pleural fluid in the order of —— ml :

A. 5-10 B. 10-15
C. 15-25 D. Above 25

1023. Severe fat embolism is associated with radiological findings resembling :

A. Pulmonary Oedema B. Pleural effusion
C. Pulmonary Infarction D. All of the above.

1024. Right side of mediastinal shadow is formed by all except :

A. RV B. Left brachiocephalic vein
C. RA D. IVC

1025. Commonest posterior mediastinal mass is :

A. Neurogenic tumours B. Lymphoma
C. Pericardial cysts D. Aneurysms

Ans.	**1015. D**	**1016. A**	**1017. D**	**1018. B**	**1019. D**	**1020. D**
	1021. A	**1022. A**	**1023. A**	**1024. B**	**1025. A**	

1026. In chest X-ray, irregular calcification is because of :

A. Echinococcal cyst B. Hamartoma
C. Bronchiectasis D. Bronchial adenoma

1027. Unilateral elevation of diaphragm is commonly due to:

A. Obesity B. Large liver
C. Scoliosis D. Congenital causes

1028. Hemoptysis and haematuria, pulmonary infiltrates and nephritis suggests:

A. Uremic pneumonia B. Collagen disease
C. Good pasture's syndrome D. Hypernephroma

1029. Diagnostic sign in carcinoma lung in Chest X-ray is :

A. Rib erosion
B. Central destruction within the lesion
C. Flattening of diaphragm
D. Elevation of diaphragm

1030. Kerley lines are :

A. Lines caused by Pulmonary fibrosis in TB
B. Lines caused by increased venous channels
C. Lines to study craniovertebral junction
D. Pulmonary lymphatics dilatation in mitral stenosis

1031. In uremic lung, there is :

A. Pulmonary edema B. Fibrosis
C. Alveolar injury D. CVC liver

1032. Extramedullary hemopoiesis is usually manifested in the chest by:

A. Mediastinal mass
B. Posterior paravertebral mass
C. Cardiac enlargement
D. Hillar adenopathy.

1033. "Signet ring" and "tramlines" on CT Scan is typically seen in :

A. Saccular bronchiectasis B. Fusiform bronchiectasis
C. Varicose bronchiectasis D. Cystic bronchiectasis

1034. In Williams-Campbell syndrome, there is :

A. Structural defect of bronchi
B. Abnormal mucociliary transport
C. Abnormal secretions
D. 1-antitrypsin deficiency

1035. Popcorn calcification in chest X-ray is seen in :

A. Sarcoidosis B. Hamartoma
C. Legionella pneumonia D. Congenital cyst

Ans.	1026. B	1027. C	1028. C	1029. A	1030. D	1031. A
	1032. B	1033. B	1034. A	1035. B		

1036. A hematoma of lung following truama present as :
A. A cyst
B. Atelectasis
C. Fleural fluid
D. Pneumonitis

1037. Honey-comb lung is seen in which of the following neurocutaneous syndrome ?
A. von Recklinghausen's
B. Sturge-Weber
C. Tuberous sclerosis
D. Von Hippel-Lindau

1038. Early change of pulmonary edema in chest X-ray :
A. Batswing appearance
B. Pleural effusion
C. Kerley B lines
D. Ground glass lung field

1039. Commonest cause of chylothorax is :
A. Trauma
B. Filariasis
C. Neoplasm
D. Idiopathic

1040. Commonest presentation of chronic coccidio-domycosis is :
A. Haemoptysis
B. Hilar lymphadenopathy
C. Patchy infiltrates in lower lobes
D. Asymptomatic

1041. In right sided chest X-ray, (PA view), hilum is formed by following except :
A. Sup. lobe vein
B. Inf. lobe vein
C. Proximal bronchi
D. Pulmonary artery

1042. Chickenpox pneumonia is characterised by:
A. Nodular infiltrate
B. Basilar infiltrate
C. Linear fibrotic pattern
D. Pulmonary oedema pattern.

1043. Both superior and inferior suface of the rib notching is seen in :
A. Coarctation of Arota
B. Superior vena caval obstruction
C. Neurofibromatosis
D. Hyperparathyroidism.

1044. Spot out wrong statement against interstitial pulmonary oedema :
A. Kerley's A lines are present
B. Kerley's B lines are present
C. Perihilar haze
D. Vascular marking becomes clear and prominent

1045. Coin shadows in chest can be better visualised in :
A. Erect penetrating P.A. view of chest
B. Tomography
C. Supine A.P. View of chest
D. Lateral view of chest.

1046. Solitary nodule in lung cannot be:
A. Tuberculoma
B. Neurofibroma
C. Bronchogenic carcinoma
D. Lymphoma

Ans.	**1036. A**	**1037. C**	**1038. C**	**1039. C**	**1040. A**	**1041. C**
	1042. B	**1043. C**	**1044. A**	**1045. B**	**1046. D**	

1047. The characteristic X-ray feature of pancoast tumour is :

A. Coin shadow
B. Apical consolidation
C. Apical mass lesion with erosion of neck of 1 & 2 ribs
D. Hilar mass

1048. Jug handle appearance of chest is seen in:

A. TOF B. MR
C. Pericardial effusion D. PAH

1049. Following are true about histoplasmosis except :

A. Mediastinal widening
B. Miliary spread to other areas of lung
C. Calcified lesions
D. None of the above

1050. "Grape-skin" thin-walled cavities are seen in :

A. TB
B. Castleman's disease
C. Williams-Campbell syndrome
D. Coccidioidomycosis

1051. "Bulging fissure" patten of pneumonia is seen with:

A. Streptococcu B. Klebsiella
C. Staph. aureus D. Varicella

1052. Incidence of pulmonary metastasis is maximum with:

A. Choriocarcinoma B. Wilm's tumor
C. Ewing's tumor D. Seminoma

1053. Mass within a cavity be seen in all except:

A. Mycetoma B. Abscess
C. Hydatid cyst D. Squamous cell carcinoma

1054. Which is the commonest form of subphrenic abscess:

A. Raised hemidiaphragm.
B. Basal consolidation
C. Pleural effusion
D. Subdiapragmatic calcification.

1055. Right sided pleural effusion may be seen in all except :

A. CHF
B. Pancreatitis
C. Budd Chiari syndrome
D. Transection of proximal thoracic duct.

1056. Ground glass appearance is not seen in :

A. Hyaline membrane disease B. Pneumonia
C. Left to right shunt D. Obstructive TAPVC

Ans.	**1047. C**	**1048. D**	**1049. D**	**1050. D**	**1051. B**	**1052. A**
	1053. D	**1054. A**	**1055. C**	**1056. C**		

1057. Multiple pleural densities are more often due to:
A. Thyomoma B. Loculated pleural effusion
C. Mesothelioma D. Metastasis

1058. Commonest malignant tumour of chest wall in children is:
A. Neuroblastoma B. Ewing sarcoma
C. Rhabdomiosarcoma D. Lymphosarcoma

1059. Cavitatory lesions in lung are seen in following except :
A. Malignant melanoma B. Ca cervix
C. Renal cell carcinoma D. Osteosarcoma

1060. In A 2 year child, true about thymus are following except:
A. Widening of mediastinum on X-ray
B. Shift of trachea
C. Steriod reduce the size
D. Sharp border with snail like appearance

1061. Continuous diaphragm is seen in :
A. Pneumomediastinum B. Pneumoperitoneum
C. Pneumoopericardium D. Pleural effusion

1062. The following can be features of calcification of benign solitary pulmonary nodule except :
A. Peripheral B. Popcorn
C. Low density D. Lamellar

1063. Investigation of choice for minimal bronchiectasis is :
A. Plain X-ray chest B. Bronchography
C. Ultrasound chest D. CT scan chest

1064. A 56 yr old made pt. was found to have s 5 cm cavity in the left apex, the age of which was not known, the next investigation to be done is :
A. CT
B. Bronchoscopy with brushings with biopsy
C. Bronchography
D. Percutaneus needle aspiration

1065. In chest trauma , immediate x-ray shows opaque shadow. The diagnosis is:
A. Haemothorax B. Pulmonary contusion
C. Pneumothorax D. Pericardial effusion

1066. Hypertranslucency of lung unilaterally is seen in all except :
A. Pneumothorax B. Resection of mammary gland
C. Pulm art. obstruction D. Pneumonectomy

1067. In pulm. embolism, findings in perfusion scan is :
A. Perfusion segmental defect

Ans.	1057. C	1058. B	1059. D	1060. D	1061. A	1062. A
	1063. B	1064. B	1065. B	1066. C	1067. A	

B. Perfusion defect with normal lung scan & radiography
C. Tenting of diaphragm
D. Normal chest scan

1068. All of the following indicate malignancy in chest X-ray except
A. Pleural effusion
B. Calcification of lesion
C. Mediastinal widening
D. Eccentric cavity

1069. Regarding tuberculosis which one is true :
A. Cavity indicates active infection
B. Peripheral rim of ring enhancement of involved lobe suggest active infection
C. Calcification indicates healed disease
D. Commonly associated with basal lesion

1070. Unilateral hyperinflation of lung is seen in :
A. Collapse
B. Congenital lobar emphysema
C. Bronchiectasis
D. Ca lung

1071. All of the following cause miliary shadow on X-ray chest except :
A. Tuberculosis
B. Histoplasmosis
C. Coccidiodomycosis
D. Wegener granulomatosis

1072. X-ray picture in hyaline membrane disease :
A. Soap bubble appearance
B. Honey limb appearance
C. Reticular granulates appearance
D. None

1073. More of lower lobe lesions are seen in :
A. TB
B. Silicosis
C. Asbestosis
D. CF

1074. Bat wing appearance of CXR is due to :
A. Cardiogenic pulmonary edema
B. TB plural effusion
C. Meig's syndrome
D. Bronchogenic carcinoma

1075. On x-ray examination of a solitary pulmonary nodule which of the following favors a benign nature :
A. Eccenteric calcification
B. Bulls eye calcification
C. Lesion is associated with atelectasis
D. Associated with pleural effusion

Ans.	1068. B	1069. D	1070. B	1071. D	1072. C	1073. C
	1074. A	1075. B				

1076. Residual mediastinal/retroperitoneal lymphoma is best assessed by :

A. Gallium scan B. Tech-99m pyrophosphate
C. Restaging procedure D. Bipedal lymphangiography

1077. Air crescent sign on X-ray chest is s/in :

A. Lung abscess B. Adenoma lung
C. Aspergilloma D. TB

1078. Bedford's sign is :

A. Splaying of carinal angle
B. Elevation of left main-stem bronchus
C. Leftward shifting of aorta
D. Seen in left ventricular enlargement

1079. A young man with pulmonary tuberculosis presents with massive recurrent hemoptysis. For angiographic treatment, which vascular structure should be evaluated first?

A. Pulmonary artery B. Bronchial artery
C. Pulmonary vein D. Superior venacava

1080. A 55 year old man who has been on bed rest for the past 10 days, complains of breathlessness and chest pain. The chest x-ray is normal. The next step in investigation should be?

A. Lung Ventilation - perfusion scan
B. Pulmonary arteriography
C. Pulmonary venous wedge angiography
D. Echocardiography

1081. From lung to tissues O_2 transported is :

A. 70% B. 86%
C. 91% D. 97%

1082. In an normal adult, the ratio of physiological and anatomical dead space is :

A. 2 : 1 B. 1 : 3
C. 3 : 1 D. 1 : 1

1083. In a normal adult, 24 hour production of CO_2 is about :

A. 150 L B. 280 L
C. 330 D. 410 L

1084. Consider the following statements :
Periodic (Cheyne-Stokes) breathing is seen

1. After voluntary apnoea
2. After voluntary hyperpnoea
3. At high altitude
4. During wakeful states of adult human being

Of these statements :

A. 1 and 2 are correct B. 3 and 3 are correct
C. 2, 3 and 4 are correct D. 1, 3 and 4 are correct

Ans.	**1076. D**	**1077. C**	**1078. A**	**1079. B**	**1080. A**	**1081. B**
	1082. D	**1083. B**	**1084. A**			

1085. Muscles of inspiration include which of the following ?

A. Diaphragm and internal intercostals
B. Diaphragm and abdominal muscles
C. Abdominal muscles and external intercostals
D. Diaphragm and external intercostals

1086. Max mid exp. flow rate-indicates flow obstruction in :

A. Large airways B. Small airways
C. Trachea D. Trachea & bronchi

1087. Respiratory minute volume in a normal person :

A. 1.2 L/min B. 2.1 L/min
C. 4.2 L/minD. 6.0 L/min

1088. In sternuous exerise, PO_2 (mmHg) falls from :

A. 40 to 1 B. 60 to 35
C. 25 to 10 D. 35 to 0

1089. During exercise, O_2 entering the blood may increase from 250 ml/ min at to rest as high as :

A. 4 L/miB. 10 L/min
C. 20 L/minD. 30 L/min

1090. The point at which breathing can no longer be voluntarily inhibited is called :

A. Herring Breuer refle B. Breaking point
C. Saturation pointD. Any of the above

1091. The stimulatory effects of hypoxia on ventilation do not clearly manifest until they become enough to override the counterbalancing inhibitory effects of a decline in :

A. Arterial H^+ B. Arterial H^+ and PCO_2
C. Venous H^+ D. PO_2

1092. There is no stimulation of ventilation by hypoxia until the alveolar PO2 falls below :

A. 60 mm HgB. 58 mm Hg
C. 50 mm Hg D. 45 mm Hg

1093. Stimuli affecting respiratory centre include :

A. CO_2 and O_2 B. Proprioceptors
C. Baroreceptors D. All of the above

1094. Carbon dioxide affects respiratory centre via :

A. Aortic bodies
B. Carotid bodies
C. Inflation and deflation receptors
D. CSF H^+ concentration

Ans.	1085. D	1086. B	1087. B	1088. A	1089. A	1090. B
	1091. B	1092. A	1093. D	1094. D		

1095. The respiratory minute volume is proportionate to the metabolic rate and the link between metabolism and ventilation is :

A. CO_2 B. O_2
C. Proteins D. All of the above

1096. Of the approximately 49 ml of CO2 in each dl of arterial blood, the quantity of dissolved, carbamino compounds and in HCO3 form is :

	Dissloved	Carbamino	Compounds HCO3-
A.	2.6 ml	2.6 ml	43.8 ml
B.	43.8 ml	2.6 ml	2.6 ml
C.	43.8 ml	3.7 ml	0.4 ml
D.	2.6 ml	43.8 ml	3.7 ml

1097. Which is untrue about chloride shift :

A. Essentially complete in 1 sec.
B. Chloride, content of arterial blood is more than venous blood
C. Vice versa of 'b' choice
D. Diffusion of Cl^- into the red cells

1098. The ambient pressure increases by — atmosphere for every 10 m of depth in sea water and every 10.4 of depth in fresh water :

A. 0.3 B. 0.8
C. 1.0 D. 1.8

1099. Cheyne-stokes breathing is seen in :

A. CHF B. Uremia
C. Brain D. Any of the above

1100. Hyperbaric oxygenation is useful in all except :

A. Congenital heart disease
B. Gas gangrene
C. Carbon monoxide poisoning
D. Nitrogen toxicity

1101. The Alveolar ventilation in an individual with Tidal Volume : 600 ml, Dead space 150 ml & respiratory rate - 15/min is :

A. 2 L/minB. 4.5 L/min
C. 6.75 L/minD. 9 L/min

1102. When the atmospheric pressure is halved, which of the following is not likely to develop:

A. An increase in pulmonary ventilation
B. A fall in arterial pO2
C. A rise in arterial pH
D. A rise in cerebral blood flow

Ans. **1095. A** **1096. A** **1097. C** **1098. C** **1099. D** **1100. D** **1101. C** **1102. D**

1103. Contraction of smooth muscle in respiratory tract occurs in response to all, except :

A. Irritation of bronchial mucosa
B. Stimulation of local beta adrenoceptors
C. A decrease in the pCO_2 in the bronchial air
D. A cold stimulus to the bronchial mucosa

1104. The surfactant material lining the lung alveoli :

A. Decreases the surface tension of alveolar fluid
B. Increases the compliance of lungs
C. Has increasingly less effect, the more lungs are inflated
D. Is decreased when pulmonary blood flow is inter- rupted
E. All of the above

1105. An increase in ventilation occurs in all except :

A. Fall in plasma bicarbonate
B. Sleep
C. Fall in pH of CSF
D. Rise in blood adrenaline level

1106. During the initial part of inspiration, which of the following does not occur ?

A. An intrapulmonary pressure falls
B. Intrathoracic pressure rises
C. Intrabdominal pressure rises
D. The partial pressure of O_2 in dead space rise

1107. What is not true for respiration centre ?

A. Situated in the medulla and pons
B. Sends out regular bursts of impulses to expiratory muscles during quiet respiration
C. Sends out regular impulses to expiratory muscles during quiet respiration
D. Is inhibited during swallowing and vomiting

1108. What factor determines the quantity of gas that will diffuse through a barrier?

A. Surface area available for diffusion and thickness of barrier
B. Molecular weight of diffusing particle
C. Solubility of particle in medium
D. Driving pressure
E. All of the above

1109. Apnoea means :

A. Cessation of breathing
B. Shallow breathing
C. Distressed breathing
D. Increased breathing rate

Ans. 1103. B 1104. E 1105. B 1106. B 1107. C 1108. E 1109. A

1110. Destruction of lung tissue and defective gaseous exchange causes all, except :

A. Prominent P wave
B. Decreased cerebral blood circulation
C. Increased red cell number
D. Pulmonary hypertension

1111. The diffusing capacity for carbon dioxide compared to that for oxygen is :

A. 20 times B. 10 times
C. 5 times D. 2 times

1112. At a tidal volume of 500 ml, physiological dead space 150 ml and respiratory rate 12/min. the alveolar ventilation in ml/minute is :

A. 6000 B. 4200
C. 180 D. 900

1113. Total vital capacity is decreased but timed vital capacity is normal in :

A. Bronchial Asthma B. Scoliosis
C. Chronic bronchitis D. All the above

1114. The intrapleural pressure (mm Hg) at the end of deep inspiration is :

A. -4 B. +4
C. -18 D. +18

1115. An increase in ventillation occurs in all situations except :

A. Decrease plasma HCO3- B. Sleep
C. Decreased pH in CSF D. Increased blood adrenaline

1116. When CO2 in inspired air increases beyond 10% at atmospheric pressure, it causes :

A. Decreased ventillation B. Depression of CNS
C. Diminished sensory acquity D. All of the above

1117. What occurs in acclimatization to a high altitude :

A. Hyperventillation
B. Polycythemia
C. O2 dissociation curve shifts to right
D. Decreased concentration of systemic capillaires

1118. Arterial pO2 is reduced in :

A. Anaemia
B. KCN poisoning
C. Pulmonary hypoventilation
D. CO poisoning

Ans.	1110. B	1111. A	1112. B	1113. B	1114. A	1115. B
	1116. D	1117. C	1118. C			

1119. When CO_2 is removed in the lungs, which of the following also occur :
A. Efflux of HCO_3^- from RBC B. Efflux of Cl- from RBC
C. Efflux of CO_2 D. Efflux of O_2 and influx CO_2

1120. The renal body fluid volume mechanism for regulating arterial pressure is important for :
A. Raising the pressure when a person stand suddenly after having been in a lying position
B. Minimizing a decrease in arterial pressure following severe hemorrhage
C. Increasing arterial pressure during sternuous physical exercise
D. Maintaining arterial pressure at a normal level over a period of weeks, months or years

1121. The most important substance controlling alveolar ventilation :
A. O_2B. CO_2
C. H_2O D. None of the above

1122. Surfactant is decreased or absent in :
A. Emphysema
B. Bronchial asthma
C. Respiratory Distress Syndrome (RDS) in children
D. RDS in adults

1123. CO_2 enters capillaries by :
A. Diffusion B. Permeation
C. Osmosis D. Active transport

1124. Carbon monoxide is released in lungs from :
A. Iron of hema moleculeB. Plasma
C. TransferrinD. Plasma

1125. Effort during normal respiration is done for purpose :
A. Lung elasticity B. Respiratory air passages
C. Alveolar air spaces D. Creating negative pleural pressure

1126. A person ascends to 12,000 feet, develops acute breathlessness; this is due to :
A. Decreased pulmonry blood flow
B. Carbon dioxide washout
C. Decreased hypoxic stimulation of respiration
D. Mechanical interference of thorax

1127. A patient is respiring 21/mt (Pulm. ventilation) and has respiratory rate of 20/mt. Which of the following is true :
A. Doing exercise B. Has respiratory acidosis
C. Cheyne Stokes breathing D. Respiring in dead space

1128. An increase in ventillation occurs in all except :
A. Decreased Plasma HCO3- B. Decreased pH of CSF
C. Increased Blood adrenaline D. None of the above

Ans.	1119. B	1120. D	1121. B	1122. C	1123. A	1124. C
	1125. A	1126. B	1127. D	1128. D		

1129. Maximum voluntary ventillation (L/min) is :

A. 90-120 B. 125-170
C. 170-210 D. 210-250

1130. CO2 influences respiration by acting at :

A. Cerebrum B. Carotid body
C. Whole of Medulla D. Respiratory centre

1131. Alveolar ventillation (L/mt) at rest is :

A. 3. B 4.2
C. 6 D. 125

Match the following :

A. 3000 ml B. 4600 ml
C. 500 ml D. 3500 ml

1132. Tidal volume
1133. Inspiratory reserve volume
1134. Vital capacity
1135. Inspiratory capacity

1136. The substance synthesized or stored in lung tissue and released into blood :

A. Histamine B. Kalikrein
C. Prostoglandins E and F D. All of the above

1137. FRC comprises of :

A. Dead space volume
B. Residual volume
C. Volume of air present after normal expiration
D. Volume which can be inhaled after normal inspiration

1138. Surfactant is secreted by :

A. Pneumocyte I B. Pneumocyte II
C. Goblet cells D. Pulmonary vessels

1139. Spirometry measures all of the following except :

A. Tidal volum B. Vital capacity
C. FEV1 D. None of the above

1140. Normal value of FEV1 in an adult male is :

A. 95% B. 80%
C. 65% D. 50%

1141. Oxygen toxicity limits exposures to less than —— hours and pressures to — atmosphres or less respectively :

A. 3, 5 B. 5, 3
C. 1, D. 2, 1

1142. At 3000 m above sea level, PO2 is about :

A. 70 mm Hg B. 60 mm Hg
C. 50 mm Hg D. 45 mm Hg

Ans.						
	1129. B	1130. D	1131. B	1132. C	1133. A	1134. B
	1135. D	1136. D	1137. C	1138. B	1139. D	1140. B
	1141. B	1142. B				

1143. As one ascends higher than 3000 m sea level, there is :

	PO2	PCO2
A.	Decrease	Increase
B.	Decrease	Decrease
C.	Increase	Increase
D.	Increase	Decrese

1144. Air in the pleural cavity causes all, except :
A. Reduction in residual volume
B. Abnormal dullness to percussion of the affected side
C. Less obvious rib contours on the affected side
D. Reduced vital capacity

1145. Circulation time through pulmonary capillaries is :
A. Less than 1 sec B. 10 sec
C. 20 sec D. 30 sec

1146. Pulmonary venules are constricted by the following except :
A. 5 HT B. Histamine
C. E. Coli endotoxin D. Isoproterenol

1147. If respiratory rate is 10/min, the alveolar ventillation is 4500 ml, and when respiratory rate becomes 30/min the alveolar ventilation will be
A. 500 mlB. 1000 ml
C. 1500 mlD. 4500 ml

1148. FEV1/FVC is reduced to :
A. Asthma B. Pleural effusion
C. Fibrosis D. All of the above

1149. Total dead space can be calculated from :
A. PCO2 of expired air
B. PCO2 of alveolar gas
C. Tidal volume
D. All of the above

1150. Diffusion capacity of lungs for O2 at rest in ml/min/mm Hg is :
A. 5 B. 10
C. 20 D. 50

1151. In health, physiologic dead space is :
A. Double than that of anatomic dead space
B. Less than that of anatomic dead space
C. Triple than that of anatomic dead space
D. Equal

1152. In cigarette smoking, surfactant is :
A. Increased
B. Decreased
C. Increased followed by decrease
D. Unlatered

Ans.	1143. B	1144. B	1145. A	1146. D	1147. C	1148. A
	1149. D	1150. C	1151. D	1152. B		

1153. Inspiratory capacity is total of :

A. Residual volume (RV) + Inspiratory reserve volume (IRV)
B. IRV + TV
C. IRV + ERV
D. ERV + RV

1154. Inspiratory capacity is :

A. 3.8 litres in women B. 3.3 litres in women
C. 2.4 litres in women D. 1.8 litres in women

1155. Functional residual capacity in a male is :

A. 3. 8 litres B. 3.3 litres
C. 2.8 litres D. 2. 2 litres

1156. Timed vital capacity in 1 sec is :

A. 73 % B. 83%
C. 87% D. 97%

1157. Work done in quiet breathing is :

A. 0.1 Kg-m/min B. 0.2 Kg-m/min
C. 0.5 Kg-m/minD. 2.5 Kg-m/min

1158. Maximum work of breathing is :

A. 0.5 Kg-m/breath B. 2.0 Kg-m/breath
C. 5.0 Kg-m/breath D. 10 Kg-m/breath

1159. Which of the following volume is equal in both men and women:

A. Inspiratory reserve volume B. Tidal volume
C. Residual volume D. Vital capacity

1160. Vital capacity in men is :

A. 4.2 litres B. 4.8 litres
C. 6.0 litres D. 6.8 litres

1161. There are about :

A. 50 million alveoli in man B. 100 million alveoli in man
C. 300 million alveoli in man D. 500 million alveoli in man

1162. The total area of the alveolar walls in contact with capillaries in both lungs is about :

A. 10 sq. mB. 30 sq. m
C. 70 sq. mD. 120 sq. m

1163. Tidal volume in both men and women is :

A. 250 ml B. 500 ml
C. 1000 ml D. 1200 ml

1164. Times vital capacity in 3 sec is :

A. 83% B. 87%
C. 97%D. 99.9 %

Ans.	1153. B	1154. C.	1155. D	1156. B	1157. C	1158. D
	1159. B	1160. B	1161. C	1162. C	1163. B	1164. C

1165. The following active substances are metabolized by the lung :

A. Kallikrein
B. Serotonin
C. Angiotonsin I —> Angiotensin II
D. All of the above

1166. The blood in the systemic arteries which bypass the pulmonary capillaries is about :

A. 0% B. 2%
C. 10% D. 15%

1167. Pulmonary blood volume increases by upto :

A. 50 ml in a normal individual when he lies down
B. 100 ml in a normal individual when he is lies down
C. 200 ml in a normal individual when he lies down
D. 400 ml in a normal individual when he lies down

1168. Pulmonary arterioles are constricted by the following except :

A. Norepinephrine B. Epinephrine
C. Angiotensin II D. Acetylcholine

1169. Respiratory quotient of cerebral tissue is :

A. 0.75-0.95 B. 0.95-0.99
C. 1.0-1.1 D. 1.1-1.2

1170. A man breathes about :

A. 100 ml of air per breath B. 250 ml of air per breath
C. 500 ml of air per breath D. 1000 ml of air per breath

1171. CO_2 which is excreted per minute is :

A. 50 ml B. 100 ml
C. 200 ml D. 400 ml

1172. In a healthy adult, 24 hour production of CO2 is about :

A. 120 litres B. 250 litres
C. 330 litres D. 410 litres

1173. The percentage of oxygen transported from the lung to the tissues in chemical combination is :

A. 28 B. 75
C. 89 D. 97

1174. The volume of gas contained in the lung at the end of maximum inspiration is :

A. Functional residual capcity
B. Inspiratory capacity
C. Inspiratory reserve volume
D. Total lung capacity

Ans. **1165. D** **1166. B** **1167. D** **1168. D** **1169. B** **1170. C**
1171. C **1172. C** **1173. D** **1174. D**

1175. Diffusion capacity of lungs for carbon monoxide is :

A. 0-5 ml/min/mmHg B. 5-10 ml/min/mmHg

C. 10-30 ml/min/mmHg D. 40-80 ml/min/mmHg

1176. Timed vital capacity in 2 sec is :

A. 83%B. 87%

C. 94%D. 97%

1177. Anatomical dead space is :

A. 50-100 mlB. 100-250 ml

C. 250-400 mlD. 400-500 ml

1178. Hearing Breuer reflex :

A. Initiates the rhythmicity of normal breathing

B. Influences only the depth of normal breathing

C. Influences depth and rate of normal breathing

D. All of these

E. Both b+c

1179. Cheyne stroke respiration is characterized by :

A. Continuous hyperpnoea

B. Increased sensitivity of resp. center

C. Fluctuating PO2 and stable PCO2

D. Decreased sensitivity of resp. center

E. Normal circulation time from lung to brain

1180. More resistance in expiration is due to :

A. Airflow during expiration

B. Compression of airway

C. Change from linear to turbulent flow

D. Saturation with moisture

1181. Three week residence at 4000 m altitude may result in :

A. Metabolic acidosi B. Metabolic alkalosis

C. Respiratory acidosisD. Respiratory alkalosis

1182. Arterial blood gas analysis in carbon monoxide poisoning is :

A. PO_2 normal, O_2 saturation less

B. PO_2 less, O_2 saturation normal

C. PO_2 less, O_2 saturation decreased

D. PO_2 less, O_2 saturation normal

1183. Which gas is not responsible for Green House effect :

A. Carbon dioxide B. Ozone

C. Nitrogen D. Nitrous oxide

1184. Peak expiratory flow rate is :

A. 5 L/mt B. 20 L/mt

C. 50 L/mt D. 400-500 L/mt

Ans.	**1175. C**	**1176. C**	**1177. B**	**1178. A**	**1179. B**	**1180. B**
	1181. D	**1182. A**	**1183. D**	**1184. D**		

1185. When vagus nerve is severed, the respiration is :

A. DecreasedB. Increased
C. CeasedD. No change

1186. When dead space is ↑, it affects alveolar :

A. PCO2 B. PO2
C. Both PCO2 and PO2 D. Neither PCO2 nor PO2

1187. Contraction of which of the following muscles is most important for causing forceful expiration :

A. Internal intercostals B. Diaphragm
C. External intercostals D. Abdominals

1188. The major cause of the hyperpnea of muscular exercise is :

A. Stimulation of the respiratory centre by the cerebral cortex and the joint proprioception
B. Hypercapnia
C. Hypoxemia
D. Alkalosis
E. Peripheral chemoreceptors

1189. If a person has a tidal volume of 411 ml, physiological dead space volume of 100 ml. and a respirtory minute ventilation of 360 ml/min., what is his alveloar ventilation :

A. 3600 ml/min B. 3000 ml/min
C. 2700 ml/min D. 1500 ml/min

1190. The major factor regulating alveolar ventilation during rest is :

A. Arterial PO2
B. Arterial PCO2
C. Arterial pH
D. Nervous output from the joint proprioceptor

1191. Which of the following does not occur in high altitude acclimatisation :

A. Reticulocytosis
B. Increase serum erythropoietin
C. Increased serum cortisol
D. Increased blood glucose

1192. Rise of pulmonary arterial pressure is caused by :

A. Hypoxia B. Acidosis
C. Alkalosis D. All of the above

1193. A swimmer breathing through a snorkel has a respiration rate of 10/min., a tidal volume of 550 ml and an effective anatomic dead space of 250 ml. What is his alveolar ventilation rate :

A. 2500 ml/min.B. 3000 ml/min.
C. 3500 ml/min.D. 4000 ml/min.

Ans.	1185. A	1186. B	1187. D	1188. A	1189. C	1190. B
	1191. D	1192. A	1193. B			

1194. The tidal volume can never become greater than the :

A. Anatomic dead space
B. Vital capacity
C. Functional residual capacity
D. Residual volume
E. Inspiratory capacity

1195. The partial pressure of oxygen in the arterial blood is normally lower than that of the alveolar gas primarily because :

A. Blood move through the lungs too fast
B. Oxygen requires a pressure gradient to diffuse into blood
C. Some portions of the lungs are ventilated but not perfused
D. Some portions of the lungs are perfused but not ventilated

1196. In the tissues, the pCO2 remains normally :

A. Of the order of 50 mmHg B. Of the order of 40 mmHg
C. Of the order of 100 mmHg D. Above 100 mmHg

1197. In respiratory alkalosis :

A. The plasma bicarbonate concentration is either low or normal
B. The cerebral blood flow increases
C. The urine is acidic
D. All of the above

1198. All of the following statements about the residual volume are true except :

A. It is the volume of gas hat remains in the lung after a maximal expiration
B. It averages 4-5 litres in a 70-kg adult male
C. It may be measured by an indicator dilution technique
D. It increases with age

W.1199. During inspiration, the :

A. Heart rate tends to decrease
B. Jugular venous pressure tends to fall
C. Muscles of the anterior abdominal wall relax
D. Intrapulmonary pressure falls below the intrapleural pressure

1200. Best airway measurement is :

A. FEV B. FEV1
C. Vital capacity D. Inspiratory Reserve volume

Match the values of pressure listed below with the appropriate arterial and venous gases :

A. 20 mm Hg B. 40 mm Hg
C. 45 mm Hg D. 100 mm Hg
E. 569 mm Hg

Ans.	1194. B	1195. D	1196. C	1197. A	1198. B	1199. B,C
	1200. B					

1201. Arterial pO_2

1202. Venous pCO_2

1203. Arterial pCO_2 and venous pO_2

1204. The parital pressure of water vapor in the lungs :

A. Increases with hyperventilation
B. Is relatively constant with changes in altitude
C. Is proportional to the CO2 concentration
D. Becomes negative when barometric pressure falls below 47 mm Hg

1205. Mucociliary action of upper respiratory tract is :

A. Protective function
B. Is of no physiological importance
C. Hinders inspiration
D. Increases the velocity of inspired air

1206. Hyperpnoea in exercise is because of :

A. Hypercapnoea
B. Hypoxaemia
C. Reflex
D. Stimulation of cortex and proprioceptors

1207. Alveolar hyperventillation causes :

A. Respiratory acidosis B. Respiratory alkalosis
C. Metabolic acidosis D. Metabolic alkalosis

1208. Normally, insensible water loss through respiratory tract and skin per day is:

A. 600-800 ml B. 100-200 ml
C. 250-300 ml D. > 1000 ml

1209. Pulmonary wedge pressure corresponds to :

A. Right atrial pressure B. Right ventricular pressure
C. Left atrial pressure D. Left ventricular pressure

1210. If the RR is 10/min Tidal vol. - 600 ml and min. volume - 6 L; alveolar ventillation is :

A. 4500 ml B. 6000 ml
C. 3600 ml D. 9000 ml

1211. True about decrease in respiration is :

A. Stops during swallowing B. Asphyxia
C. Hypoxic hypoxia D. Paradoxical respiration

1212. Respiratory centre controlled by Pons is :

A. Gasping B. Pneumotaxic
C. Inspiratory D. Expiratory

1213. FeV2/FeV less than 60% is seen in :

A. Emphysema B. Rectus excavatum
C. Interestitial lung disease D. Pulmonary oedema

Ans.							
	1201. D	1202. C	1203. B	1204. B	1205. A	1206. B	1207. B
	1208. A	1209. C	1210. A	1211. A	1212. B	1213. A	

1214. In Interstitial lung disease, not seen is :

A. ↑ pO_2 in blood
B. ↑ pCO_2 in blood
C. Response to O_2 therapy
D. FeV2/FeV are decreased in same ratio

1215. Air taken in and out per breath is :

A. Tidal volume
B. Vital capacity
C. Alveolar ventilation
D. FEV

1216. Oxygen debt :

A. Is impossible to incur when breathing pure Oxygen
B. Can never occur in healthy individual
C. Is often evidenced by an increase in lactic concentration in the blood
D. Is caused by lack of anaerobic metabolism

1217. The most important factor that tends to collapse the lungs (the recoil tendency) is the :

A. Elastic fibre in the lungs
B. Intrapleural fluid pressure
C. Total intrapleural pressure
D. Surface tension of the alveolar fluid
E. Tension in the intercostal muscles

1218. Oxygen therapy has significant value in all the following types of hypoxia except :

A. Atmospheric hypoxia
B. Hypoventilation hypoxia
C. Hypoxia due to pulmonary edema
D. Hypoxia due to decreased hemoglobin in the blood
E. Hisotoxic hypoxia due to cyanide poisoning

1219. Most potent respiratory stimulant is :

A. Oxygen
B. Carbon dioxide
C. H+
D. K+

1220. Which of the following condition is having an elevated arterial pCO2 value :

A. ARDS
B. Fat embolism
C. Pulmonary oedema
D. Emphysema

1221. The partial pressure of oxygen in the arterial blood is normally lower than that of the alveolar gas primarily because :

A. The lungs use oxygen
B. Blood moves through the lungs fast
C. Some portions of the lungs ar ventilated but not perfused
D. Some portions of the lungs are perfused but not ventilated

Ans. 1214. C 1215. A 1216. C 1217. D 1218. E 1219. B 1220. D 1221. D

1222. Compensatory responses to metbolic acidosis include all except :

A. Hyperventilation
B. An increase in titrable acid excretion
C. An increase in NH excretion
D. An increase in glycolysis by H+ activation of phosphofructokinase

1223. Respiratory movements are associated with (and partly, cause) fluctuations in blood pressure. The highest rise of systolic pressure occurs at the time of the :

A. Late inspiration-early expiration
B. End of expiration
C. Beginning of inspiration
D. Late expiration-early inspiration

1224. Structures through which O_2 must diffuse in passing from alveolar lumen to Hb :

A. Surfactant containing liquid
B. Alveolar membrane, basement membrane
C. Capillary endothelium, plasma and R.B.C. membrane
D. All of the above

1225. A total vital capacity of loss than 80% of predicted values indicate :

A. Respiratory center damage
B. Restrictive pulmonary disease
C. Metabolism is depressed
D. Obstructed air passages

1226. The majority of observers can only detect cyanosis when the arterial oxygen saturation falls below :

A. 70%B. 80%
C. 85%D. 90%

1227. When gases flow through an orifice, the factor least likely to affect the turbulance is the :

A. Viscosity of the gasB. Density of the gas
C. Pressure of the gasD. Diameter of the orifice

1228. Normal partial pressure of oxygen in arterial blood in health at sea level :

A. 60-100 mmHg B. 60-80 mmHg
C. 80-100 mmHgD. 100-200 mmHg

1229. Normal arterial oxygen concentration :

A. 100% B. 95-98%
C. 90-95% D. 80-85%

1230. Respiratory alkalosis occurs in :

A. Diabetic ketoacidosis B. Pyloric stenosis
C. Primary aldosteronism D. Excessive ventilation

Ans.	1222. D	1223. B	1224. D	1225. D	1226. B	1227. C
	1228. C	1229. B	1230. D			

1231. Respiratory acidosis is characterized by :

A. ↓ plasma HCO_3 ↓ pCO_2

B. ↑ pCO_2, ↓ pH

C. ↓ pH and ↓ pCO_2

D. ↑ pCO_2, ↑ pH

1232. Which of the following tends to decrease with age :

A. Vital capacity
B. Systolic B.P.
C. Pulse pressure
D. Residual volume

1233. Decreased FEV_1 and increased Tidal volume is seen in :

A. Emphysema
B. COAD
C. Br. asthma
D. TB

1234. Oxygen dissociation curve shifts to right in :

A. Hyperkalamia
B. Hypokalamia
C. Metabolic alkalosis
D. Anemia

1235. Commonest cause of Cheyne-stokes breathing is :

A. Contusion of the brain

B. Destructive disease of the brain

C. Increased intracranial tension

D. Cardiac failure

1236. A case of restrictive lung disease differs from obstructive lung disease in having a lower :

A. Residual volume
B. Vital capacity
C. Total lung capacity
D. All of the above

1237. True about respiratory center :

A. Continuously sends stimulatory impulses to exp. muscles

B. Has got connection with cardiac center

C. Inhibited by swallowing and vomiting

D. Directly stimulated by ↓ PaO_2

1238. Aerobic capacity is increased by :

A. Regular 3 months exercise

B. Prolonged exercise routine

C. Spurts of exercise

D. Sternous exercise

1239. Following lung volumes are measured in laboratory examination except :

A. FEV
B. Tidal volume
C. Residual volume
D. Vital capacity

1240. Hyperventilation occurs due to all of the following except :

A. Decrease in pH of CSF

B. Increase in circulating catecholeamines

C. CO poisoning

D. Aspirin poisoning

Ans.	1231. B	1232. A	1233. A	1234. D	1235. D	1236. D
	1237. C	1238. A	1239. C	1240. C		

1241. Anemic hypoxia is characterized by :

A. Low arterial pO_2
B. Low arterial O_2 content
C. Cyanosis
D. Decreased blood flow

1242. Severe hypoxia may produce :

A. BP rise
B. BP fall
C. BP Fall followed by BP rise
D. No change

1243. Dyspneic index = % breathing reserve (MVV-Maximum Voluntary ventillation, RMV-Resp. minute volume) :

A. $\frac{\text{MMV-RMV}}{\text{MVV}} \times 100$

B. $\frac{\text{(MVV-RMV)-2}}{\text{MVV}} \times 100$

C. $\frac{\text{RMV+MVV}}{\text{RMV}} \times 100$

D. $\frac{\text{MVV - RMV}}{\text{RMV}} \times 100$

1244. A patient with impaired ability to excrete CO_2 is likely to have all, except :

A. A raised blood bicarbonate level
B. An acid urine
C. A lowered arterial blood PO_2 when breathing air at atmospheric pressure
D. Cool extremities

1245. Patients with restrictive lung diseases differ from those with obstructive airways disease by having :

A. Lower ratio of forced expiratory volume in one second/vital capacity
B. Lower peak flow rate
C. Lower residual volume and total lung capacity
D. All of the above

1246. The instrument used for measuring the vital capacity and FEV is :

A. Wright peak flow meter
B. Vitalograph
C. Carlen's catheter
D. None of the above

1247. About 90% of the CO_2 entering the blood is carried as :

A. Dissolved CO_2B.
Carbonic anhydrase
C. Carbamino CO_2
D. Carbonic acid
E. Bicarbonate

Ans.	1241. B	1242. A	1243. A	1244. D	1245. C	1246. B
	1247. E					

1248. Normal adult lung weighs :

A. 100-200 g B. 200-300 g

C. 300-400 g D. 500-600 g

1249. Angular acceleration while flying may result in a pilot :

A. Hypotension B. Unconsciaisness

C. Vertebral fractures D. All of the above

1250. Initiation of respiration is done by :

A. Dorsal respiratory group B. Pneumotaxis centre

C. Nucleus parabrachialis D. Ventral respiratory group

1251. Normal PaO_2 (mmHg) is :

A. 40-60 B. 80-108

C. 60-80 D. 110-120

1252. At inspiration, the pleural pressure is :

A. More positive B. Zero

C. More negative D. Atmospheric

1253. The difference between amount of O_2 entering body (ml per min) and CO_2 excreted (ml/min) is ——— ml/min :

A. 20 B. 50

C. 0 D. -10

1254. Ventilation/perfusion ratio is maximum in :

A. Apical region B. Middle region

C. Base D. Same all over

1255. Diffusion capacity of O_2 of lungs is —— ml/min/mmHg at brest :

A. 10 B. 20

C. 30 D. 45

1256. In physiological shunt,——— % blood bypasses pulm capillaries :

A. 0.5 B. 1

C. 2 D. 4

1257. Lung diffusion capacity is measured with :

A. CO2 B. CO

C. O2 D. H2

1258. Sympathetic stimulation on the bronchus causes :

A. Bronchial constriction

B. Increased secretion of glands into Bronchi

C. No effect

D. Bronchial Dilatation

1259. Increased alveolo-arteriolar ratio is seen in following except :

A. Right to Left shunt B. Alveolar hypoventilation

C. Diffusion decreases D. None

Ans.						
	1248. C	**1249. C**	**1250. A**	**1251. C**	**1252. C**	**1253. B**
	1254. A	**1255. B**	**1256. C**	**1257. B**	**1258. D**	**1259. C**

1260. Maximum resistance during expiration is due to :
A. Collapse of alveoli
B. Expiratory Muscular fatigue
C. Dynamic collapse of air ways
D. Breaking action of inspiratory airways

1261. False about focal Bronchoconstriction during expiration :
A. Local pulmonary Hypertension
B. ↑ respiratory effort
C. ↑ respiratory minute volume
D. None of the above

1262. J receptors when stimulated causes :
A. Increased heart rate B. Apnoea
C. Tachypnoea D. Bradypnoea

1263. Which of the following is false:
A. FEV is the fraction of total lung volume in one second
B. PEFR is maximum expiratory flow of lung capacity
C. Respiratory minute volume is the amount of the air inspired per minute
D. MBC is the largest volume of gas can be moved into and out of lungs in one second by effort

1264. Normal PO2 in an 85-year healthy male in his room air breath is:
A. 80 B. 60
C. 45 D. 110

1265. The normal adult Vd/Vt ratio is :
A. <20 B. < 35
C. < 40 D. <50

1266. In high altitude mountain sickness, feature of pulmonary edema is :
A. Decreased pulmonary capillary permeability
B. Increased pulmonary capillary pressure
C. Normal left atrial pressure
D. Increased left ventricular back-pressure

1267. During inspiration the intrapleural pressure becomes :
A. Equal to Zero
B. More positive
C. More negative
D. Equal to atmospheric pressure

1268. pCO2 affects respiration primarily by stimulating :
A. Carotid and Aortic bodies B. Pulmonary 'J' receptors
C. Medullary chemoreceptors D. Barroreceptors

Ans.	1260. D	1261. C	1262. C	1263. D	1264. A	1265. C
	1266. B	1267. C	1268. C			

1269. About $\alpha 1$ antitrypsin true is :

A. Deficiency in lung causes increased compliance

B. Deficiency causes decreased elastase enzyme

C. In smokers with deficiency have increased destruction of lungs

D. All of the above

1270. Which of the following is most useful test in idiopathic pulmonary fibrosis :

A. FEV1/FVC B. VC

C. MEP D. RV

1271. Nitrogen washout method is mainly used to measure :

A. ERV B. FEFR

C. V D. FRC

1272. Following lung volume may be normal emphysema except :

A. TLC B. MEP

C. FEV1/FVC D. FEFR

1273. CO inhibits respiratory chain by A/E :

A. Binding with oxygen

B. Binding with haemoglobin

C. Producing hypoxia

D. Producing carboxyhemoglobin

1274. Sudden cessation of respiration at terminal stage shows :

A. Dynamic compression of airway

B. Collapsed alveoli

C. Expiratory muscle fatigue

D. Breaking action of insipiratory muscle

1275. In voluntary hyperventilation, muscle sprain is due to :

A. Sympathetic stimulation cause release of acetylcholine at neuro-muscular junction

B. Decrease of Ca++ in serum

C. Increase of Ca++ in serum

D. Increase actin and myosin ratio

1276. Which of the following does not affect respiration ?

A. Arterial H+ concentration

B. Arterial Na+ concentration

C. Cerebrospinal fluid CO2 concentration

D. Cerebrospinal fluid H+ concentration

1277. Which occurs after hyperventilation with 6% CO2 ?

A. Apnea

B. Continued hyperventilation

C. Cheyne-Stokes breathing

D. Kussmaul's breathing

Ans.	1269. C	1270. B	1271. D	1272. D	1273. A	1274. A
	1275. A	1276. B	1277. C			

1278. When tidal volume is 600 ml. Dead space is 150 ml and rate of respiration is 10/min., alveolar ventilation will be :

A. 4.5 litre/minB. 5.0 litre/min
C. 6.0 litre/minD. 4.0 litre/min
E. 5.5. litre/min

1279. A patient is having normal lung compliance and increased airway resistance. What is the most - economical way of breathing for him :

A. Slow and deep B. Slow and shallow
C. Rapid and deep D. Rapid and shallow

1280. A low lander goes to the mountains. When he reaches about 5,000 feet high, he develops dyspnea. Which of the following is the correct explantion for his symptom :

A. Carbon dioxide wash out
B. Increased blodo flow to the pulmonary tissues
C. CNS depression
D. Increased work of breathing

1281. Alveolar ventillation is (VC-5000 ml, PR-14/min, TV-500 ml dead space—150 ml) :

A. 4900ml B. 3500 ml
C. 2500 ml D. 6000 ml

1282. Activation of which receptor causes pulmonary vasoconstriction?:

A. Alpha 2 adrenergic B. M3 cholinergic
C. H2 histaminic D. ETa epithelial receptor

1283. In hyperventilation, muscle spasm occurs because of :

A. Increased sympathetic activity
B. Increased parasympathetic activity
C. Decreased Ca++ ions
D. Increased gamma efferent activity

1284. Bellow's spirometry measures :

A. TLC B. RV
C. Closing volume D. EERV

1285. True about 'dead space' in tracheobronchial tree is :

A. Increases in coughing
B. Humidifies air
C. Increases with adrenaline
D. In all respiratory diseases the anatomical dead space coincides with physiological dead space

1286. Pulmonary surfactant is secreted by :

A. Type I pneumocytes B. Type II pneumocytes
C. Clara cells D. Bronchial epithelial cells

Ans.	1278. A	1279. A	1280. A	1281. A	1282. D	1283. C
	1284. D	1285. B	1286. B			

1287. Poor prognostic indicator in pneumococcal pneumonia include :

A. Leucocytosis over 20000 B. Old age
C. Systemic disease D. Type II penumococcus
E. Postive blood culture

1288. Hemoptysis is important symptom in :

A. Idiopathic hemosiderosis B. Bronchial adenoma
C. Sarcoidosis D. Alpha-I-antitrypsin deficiency
E. Pulmonary T.B.

1289. Features of hypercapnia are all except :

A. Bounding pulses B. Drowsiness
C. Headache D. Cold extremities

1290. Bronchial asthma can be treated with :

A. Orciprenaline B. Aminophylline
C. Salbutamol D. Bromhexine
E. Potassium iodide

1291. Eater Lambert syndrome is seen with :

A. Oat cell carcinoma bronchus B. Myasthenia gravis
C. Thyroid cancer D. Pancreatic head cancer

1292. Pleural calcification occurs in all except :

A. Silicosis B. Asbestosis
C. Tuberculosis D. Hemothorax

1293. Tortous bronchial arteries are seen in :

A. Coarctation of aorta B. Tetralogy of Fallot
C. VSD D. ASD

1294. Sudden onset of cough followed by increasing dyspnoea is characteristic of :

A. Pleural effusion B. Lobar pneumonia
C. Myocardial infarction D. Pneumothorax

1295. Increased A.C.E. levels are diagnostic of :

A. Ca lung B. Sarcoidosis
C. Aspergillosis D. Hemosiderosis

1296. Features of Klebsiella pneumonia is/are :

A. High mortality B. Upper lobes involved
C. Systemic disturbance D. Chocolate colour sputum
E. All of the above

1297. The recent terminology for status asthmaticus is :

A. Episodic asthma B. Chronic asthma
C. Acute asthma D. Severe acute asthma

1298. Compliance of the lungs is reduced in all except :

A. Emphysema B. Pleural thickening
C. Hyaline membrane disease D. Pulmonary fibrosis

Ans.	1287. A,B,E	1288. A,B,E	1289. D	1290. A,B,C	1291. A	1292. A
	1293. A	1294. D	1295. B	1206. E	1297. D	1298. A

1299. Bovine cough is characteristic of :

A. Acute epiglottitis
B. Tracheitis
C. Laryngeal paralysis
D. Chronic laryngitis
E. Chronic bronchitis

1300. Which of the following is not a feature of Kartagener's syndrome :

A. Bronchiectasis
B. Pancreatic insufficiency
C. Sinusitis
D. Situs invertus

1301. Cyanosis and clubbing are early features of :

A. Lung abscess
B. Fibrosing alveolitis
C. Bronchogenic carcinoma
D. Sarcoidosis

1302. Shrinking lung syndrome is seen in :

A. SLE
B. Systemic solerosis
C. Polymyositis
D. Dematomyositis

1303. C-Reactive protein is not increased in :

A. Rheumatic fever
B. Active rheumatoid arthritis
C. Acute gout
D. Mumps
E. Sydenham's chorea

1304. Bronchoalveolar lavage is useful for evaluating :

A. Bronchogenic carcinoma
B. Bronchopleural histula
C. Pneumothorax
D. Interstitial lung disease

1305. Commonest cause of spontaneous pneumothorax is :

A. Rupture of sub-pleural bleb
B. T.B.
C. Trauma
D. Asthma

1306. Hamman-rich syndrome is treated with :

A. Vitamin B6
B. Vitamin B12
C. INH
D. Steroids

1307. Finger clubbing is not a usual feature with :

A. Mesothelioma
B. Bronchiectasis
C. Tropical eosinophilia
D. Fibrosing alveolitis

1308. All of the following cause pleural cavity transudation concept :

A. Empyema
B. CCF
C. Cirrhosis
D. Meig'r syndrome

1309. Earliest manifestation of pulmonary embolism is :

A. Cyanosis
B. Hemoptysis
C. Dyspnoea
D. Chest pain

1310. A patient with pulmonary tuberculosis is infectious :

A. Till sputum AFB is negative
B. Till culture negativity is confirmed
C. Till radiological opacity disappears
D. Till initial few weeks of therapy

Ans.	1299. B	1300. B	1301. B	1302. B	1303. D	1304. D
	1305. A	1306. D	1307. C	1308. A	1309. C	1310. D

1311. The following about Klebsiella pneumonia are true except :
A. Red currant jelly sputum
B. Seen in alcoholics
C. Seen in order age group
D. Penicillin is the drug of choice

1312. Pickwickian syndrome consists of :
A. Hypercapnia B. Obesity
C. Somnolence D. All of the above

1313. Alveolar hypoventilation is observed in :
A. Status asthmaticus B. Guillain Barre syndrome
C. Interstitial lung disease D. Bronchiectasis

1314. Minimum amount of sulfhemoglobin required to produce cyanosis is :
A. 0.5 gm B. 1.5 gm
C. 5 gm D. 12 gm

1315. Clubbing occurs earliest with :
A. Empyema B. Bronchiectasis
C. Cyanotic heart disease D. Crohns disease

1316. Monday dyspnea is seen with :
A. Malingering B. Pulmonary eosinophilia
C. Byssinosis D. Chronic bronchitis

1317. Post influenza bacterial infection of the lung is caused commonly by :
A. Staphylococcus B. Streptococcus
C. Pneumococcus D. Hemophilus influenzae

1318. Cyanosis may be seen in ——— poisoning :
A. Mercury B. Nitrates
C. Orgonphosphorous D. Aspirin

1319. Elevated DL co is found in :
A. Interstitial lung disease B. Emphysema
C. Pulmonary hypertension D. Alveolar hemorrhage

1320. Commonest cause of death in sarcoidosis is :
A. Pneumonia B. Corpulmonale
C. Myocardial infarction D. Liver failure

1321. Pulmonary Hemorrhage occurs in :
A. Pulmonary hypertension B. Parkinsonism
C. Cushing syndrome D. Stein Leventhal syndrome

1322. 'Creola bodies' are found in :
A. Severe bronchial asthma B. Cystic fibrosis
C. Bronchiectasis D. Aspergillosis

1323. Pink frothy expectoration is seen in :
A. Pulmonary edema B. Pulmonary tuberculosis
C. Bronchogenic carcinoma D. Mucormycosis

Ans.	1311. D	1312. D	1313. B	1314. A	1315. C	1316. C	1317. C
	1318. B	1319. D	1320. B	1321. A	1322. A	1323. A	

1324. Fungal lung infection commonly seen in diabetics is :
A. Actinomycosis B. Mucormycosis
C. Aspergillosis D. Coccidiodomycosis

1325. Crackling crepitations unaltered by coughing is characteristic of :
A. Pulmonary tuberculosis B. Interstitial lung disease
C. Klebsiella pneumonia D. Lung abscess

1326. Regarding bronchial asthma, all are bad prognostic factors except :
A. Pulsus paradoxusus B. Use of accesory muscles
C. Hyperinflated chest D. Hypocapnia

1327. Which of the following drugs are used in bronchial asthma :
A. Isoprenaline B. Salbutamol
C. Aminophylline D. All of the above

1328. Opportunistic lung infection in AIDS is due to :
A. Pneumocystis carini B. Klebsiella
C. Mucormycosis D. Mycoplasma

1329. Which of the following is not used to treat acute pulmonary edema :
A. IV fluids B. IV morphine
C. IV frusemide D. Oxygen

1330. Commonest cell type found in bronchoalveolar lavage is :
A. Macrophage B. T lymphocyte
C. B lymphocyte D. Mast cell

1331. Causes of acute pulmonary edema are all except :
A. Inhalation of irritant furnes
B. Sudden exposure to high attitudes
C. Acute left ventricular failure
D. Deep sea diving

1332. Paradoxical breathing is characteristic of :
A. Pneumonia B. Pneumothorax
C. Atelectasis D. Diaphragmatic paralysis

1333. Pleural effusion with low glucose content is characteristic of :
A. Rheumatic fever with CHF B. Rheumatoid arthritis
C. Mesothelioma D. Metapneumonic effusions

1334. Commonest source of pulmonary embolism is :
A. Iliac vein B. Femoral vein
C. Calf vein D. Inf venacava

1335. Stony dull note on percussion is characteristic of :
A. Pleural effusion B. Consolidation
C. Pleurisy D. Tuberculous cavity

1336. Tubular breathing is seen in :
A. Pleural effusion B. Consolidation
C. Pleurisy D. Tuberculous cavity

Ans.	1324. B	1325. B	1326. D	1327. D	1328. A	1329. A	1330. A
	1331. D	1332. D	1333. B	1334. A	1335. A	1336. B	

1337. Cavernous breathing is seen in :
A. Pleural effusion B. Pleural effusion
C. Consolidation D. Consolidation

1338. Tumor presenting as peripheral nodule may by :
A. Sq cell carcinoma B. Large cell carcinoma
C. Adenocarcinoma D. Small celll carcinoma

1339. Pneumatocele formation is seen in —— pneumonia :
A. Staphylococcal B. Hemophilus
C. Streptococcal D. Pneumococcal

1340. Smoking most commonly causes :
A. Carcinoma lung B. TA O
C. Chronic bronchitis D. Myocardial ischemia

1341. Amphoric breathing is seen in :
A. Pneumothorax B. Pericarditis
C. Pneumonia D. Pleural Effusion

1342. Commonest paraneoplastic syndrome associated with bronchogenic carcinoma is :
A. Hypercalcaemia B. Eaton Lambert syndrome
C. Ectopic ACTH secretion D. Nephrotic syndrome

1343. Pleural fluid low in glucose is seen in :
A. Rheumatoid arthritis B. Tuberculosis
C. Mesothelioma D. Cirrrhosis

1344. CO2 retention is seen in :
A. COPD B. Morphine administration
C. Pickwickian syndrome D. Salicylate poisoning

1345. Causes of hemorrhagic pleural effusion :
A. Pulmonary infarction B. Mesothelioma
C. Bronchial adenoma D. Tuberculosis

1346. Smallest amount of pleural fluid detectable in upright chest X-ray is :
A. 100 ml B. 175 ml
C. 250 ml D. 350. ml

1347. Volume of air taken into the lungs in normal respiration is known as :
A. Vital capacity B. Timed vital capacity
C. Tidal volume D. Inspiratory reserve volume

1348. The normal respiratory quotient is :
A. 0.5 B. 0.8
C. 0.75 D. 1.0

1349. Normal intrapleural pressure is :
A. 1 to 2 mm Hg B. 2 to 4 mm Hg
C. 0.5 to 1 mm Hg D. 3 to 4 mm Hg

Ans.	1337. C	1338. B,C		1339. A	1340. D	1341. D	1342. A
	1343. A	1344. C	1345. A	1346. B	1347. C	1348. C	1349. A

1350. Commonest cause of pleural effusion is :

A. C.C.F. B. Pheumonia

C. Malignancy D. Cirrhosis

1351. Parasites causing lung injury include :

A. Stronglyoides B. Paragonymus

C. Clonorchis D. Trichinella

1352. Silicosis causes which of the following :

A. Apical nodular fibrisosis B. Coin shadow

C. Hilar lymphadenopathy D. Basal peribrônchial fibrosis

1353. Curschmann's spirals in sputum is seen in :

A. Tuberculous cavity B. Asthma

C. Bronchitis D. Bronchiectasis

1354. Left sided pleural effusion may be found with :

A. C.C.F. B. Meig syndrome

C. Pancreatitis D. Drug induced effusion

1355. Commonest cause of bronchopleural fistula is :

A. Carcinoma bronchus B. Bronchiectasis

C. Pulmonary TB D. Bronchitis

1356. Differential cyanosis is seen in :

A. PDA with reversal of shunt B. VSD with reversal of shunt

C. Coarctation of aorta D. All of the above

1357. In Kartagener syndrome all are seen except :

A. Cystic fibrosis B. Dextrocardia

C. Sinusutus D. Absence of cilia

1358. Commonest cause of secondary pneumothorax is :

A. COPD B. Carcinoma lung

C. Pre asthma D. Lung abscess

1359. The complication least likely to occur in a case of chronic bronchitis is :

A. Pulmonary hypertension B. Pneumothorax

C. Emphysema D. Amyloidosis

1360. All are characteristic of ARDS except :

A. No response to oxygen B. Stiff lung

C. Hypercapnia D. Right to left shunt

1361. Which is not a feature of sarcoidosis :

A. Cardiomyopathy B. Malabsorption

C. Hypercalcemia D. Paratracheal lymphodes

1362. Management of choice of pneumomediastinum is :

A. Tube drainage B. Ionerdide pregnancy

C. Ventilatory support D. None of the above

Ans.	1350. A	1351. B	1352. A	1353. B	1354. C	1355. C	1356. A
	1357. A	1358. A	1359. B	1360. C	1361. A	1362. D	

1363. Hypercalcemia occurs in which type of lung cancer :
A. Oat cell B. Giant cell
C. Squamous cell D. Alveolar cell

1364. Bilateral pleural effusion is seen in :
A. Nephrotic syndrome B. Constrictive pericarditis
C. Congestive cardiac failure D. All of the above

1365. Proximal bronchiectasis, eosinophilia and asthma is seen in :
A. Aspergillosis B. Histoplasmosis
C. Nocardiosis D. Mucormycosis

1366. In Cryptogenic fibrosing alveolitis which is not seen :
A. Decreased lung capacity
B. Decreased diffusing capacity
C. Decreased arteriolar oxygen tension
D. Decreased FEV1/FVC ratio

1367. Bronchospasm is induced by :
A. Bea blockers B. Sulphonamides
C. Aspirin D. PAS

1368. Which is true regarding Eaton Lambert syndrome :
A. Guanidine gives relief
B. Neostigmine also effective
C. Ocular muscles spared
D. Associated with oat cell carcinoma

1369. Corpulmonale is seen in :
A. Marked obesity
B. Kyphoscoliosis
C. Massive pulmonary embolism
D. All

1370. Causes of hypersensitivity pneumonitis is/are :
A. Silicosis B. Farmer's lung
C. Bird fancier's lung D. Asbestosis

1371. Pulmonary embolism causes :
A. Bradycardia B. Decreased cardiac output
C. Arterial hypoxemia D. Acute right ventricular strain

1372. The following are interstitial lung diseases except :
A. Sarcoidosis B. Fibrosing alveolitis
C. Bronchial asthma D. Pneumoconiosis

1373. Sarcoidosis is charactised by all except :
A. Miliary shadow B. Pleural involvement
C. Hilar lymphadenopathy D. Egg shell calcification

Ans.						
	1363. C	**1364. D**	**1365. A**	**1366. D**	**1367. A,C**	
	1368. A,D	**1369. D**	**1370. B,C**	**1371. C,D**	**1372. C**	**1373. A**

1374. There is no correlation between X-ray appearance and clinical state of the patient in—— pneumonia :

A. Mycoplasmal B. Friedlanders
C. Pneumococal D. Staphylococcal

1375. All are features of ARDS except :

A. Pulmonary hypertension
B. Normal pulmonary artery wedge pressure
C. Hypoxemia
D. Low protein pulmonary edema

1376. All predispose to ARDS except :

A. Fat embolism B. Septicemia
C. Multiple blood transfusions D. Status asthmaticus

1377. The done of the diaphram is elevated in :

A. Typhoid fever B. Pulmonary infarction
C. Emphysema D. Bronchiectasis

1378. Alveolar hypoventilation results in :

A. Respiratory alkalosis B. Respiratory acidosis
C. Metabolic alkalosis D. Metabolic acidosis

1379. Persistent coarse crepitations in the chest is diagnostic of :

A. Pulmonary T.B. B. Cavity lesion
C. Pulmonary edema D. Bronchiectasis

1380. Commonest cause of non progresive pneumothorax is :

A. Rupture of subpleural bleb B. Tuberculosis
C. Trauma D. Bronchiectasis

1381. All are features of adult respiratory distress syndrome except :

A. Hypoxemia B. Hypercapnia
C. Pulmonary oedema D. Stiff lung

1382. Pneumothorax occurs in all except :

A. Eosinophilic granuloma
B. Marfan's syndrome
C. Assisted ventilation
D. Broncho-pulmonary aspergillosis

1383. Amyloidosis occurs in all except :

A. Tuberculosis B. Chronic bronchitis
C. Lung abscess D. Bronchiectasis

1384. All of the following are useful for treating acute bronchial asthma in children except :

A. 100% oxygen
B. Hydrocortisone infusion
C. IV aminophylline
D. Sodium chromoglycate inhalation

Ans.	1374. A	1375. B	1376. D	1377. B	1378. B	1379 D
	1380. A	1381. B	1382. A	1383. B	1384. D	

1385. The lung absces in children can be caused by all except :
A. Pneumococcus B. E. Histolytica
C. Staphylococcus D. Klebsiella

1386. 100% oxygen improves cyanosis in all except :
A. Tetralogy of Fallot B. Bronchial asthma
C. Eosinophilic pneumonia D. Interestitial lung disease

1387. Cardinal sign of respiratory arrest is :
A. Apnea B. Shallow breathing
C. Irregular breathing D. Hurried breathing

1388. Kussmaul's breathing is due to presence of :
A. Bicarbonate ions B. H+ ions
C. Chloride ions D. K+ ions

1389. Normal ventilation perfusion rate is :
A. 0.6 B. 1.0
C. 0.8 D. 1.2

1390. Normal excursion of diaphragm is :
A. 1 cm B. 3 cm
C. 4 cm D. 5 cm

1391. Maximum excursion of diaphragm is :
A. 3 cm B. 4 cm
C. 6 cm D. 8 cm

1392. Commonest Mediastinal mass is :
A. Lymphoma B. Aneurysm of aorta
C. Metastatic lymph node D. Thyroid tumour

1393. All are seen with thymic mass except :
A. Cushing syndrome B. Pure red cell
C. Myasthenia gravis D. Thrombocytopenia

1394. Pseudochylous pleural effusion is seen with :
A. Tuberculosis B. Lymphoma
C. Rheumatic Arthritis D. Trauma

1395. Contraindication of resection of bronchogenic carcinoma is :
A. Limited small cell carcinoma
B. Peripheral tumour
C. Ipsilateral lymph node
D. Invasion of carina

1396. All are correct about fat embolism except :
A. Seen 48-72 hours after injury
B. Neurological symptoms
C. Petechial hemorrhages
D. Renal shut down

Ans.						
	1385. D	1386. A	1387. A	1388. B	1389. C	1390. A
	1391. B	1392. B	1393. D	1394. A	1395. D	1396. D

1397. Commonest finding in interstitial lung disease is :
A. Rhonchi
B. Pleural rub
C. Midinspiratory crepitations
D. End inspiratory crepitations

1398. Normal Reid index is :
A. 0.2 B. 0.30
C. 0.44 D. 0.50

1399. Bulging fissures on X-ray chest is seen with :
A. Pneumococcal pneumonia
B. Kelbsiella pneumonia
C. Staph. pneumonia
D. Anaerobic infection

1400. Commonst cause of pneumoconiosis is :
A. Coal workers pneumoconiosis
B. Asbestosis
C. Silicosis
D. Bagassosis

1401. Pulmonary hemorrhage is seen with :
A. Good pastures syndrome
B. Wegeners Granulomatosis
C. Idiopathic pulmonary hemosiderosis
D. All of the above

1402. Diffusion capacity of lungs is measured by :
A. Xenon B. Carbon-Monoxide
C. Nitrogen D. Helium

1403. Most effective drug for P. carinii pneumonia is :
A. Sulfamethoxazole trimethoprim
B. Pentamidien aerosol
C. Dapsone
D. Atavaquone

1404. Most sensitive investigation for pneumococcal pneumonia is :
A. Sputum Gram staining B. Sputum culture
C. Blood culture D. Serological Tests

1405. Most sensitive test for P. carinii pneumonia is :
A. X-ray chest B. Sputum culture
C. Sputum microscopy D. Broncheoalveolar lavage

1406. Incidence of mixed infection in pneumonia is :
A. 5% B. 10%
C. 15% D. 20%

Ans.	1397. D	1398. C	1399. B	1400. B	1401. A	1402. B
	1403. A	1404. A	1405. D	1406. B		

1407. Hyperventilation is seen in all except :
A. Mitral stenosis
B. Herpes encephalitis
C. Bronchial asthma
D. Paracetamol overdosage

1408. Crepitations are seen in all except :
A. Pneumonia
B. Lung abscess
C. Bronchiolitis
D. LVLF

1409. Lung function tests are diagnostic in :
A. Asthma
B. Chronic bronchitis
C. Emphysema
D. Sarcoidosis

1410. Theophylline needs are reduced in :
A. Smokers
B. Cardiac failure
C. Cirrhosis
D. Viral infection

1411. Commonest side effect of theophylline is :
A. Tremors
B. Vomiting
C. Arrythmia
D. Convulsions

1412. Drug of choice in exercise induced asthma is :
A. Theophilline
B. Ipratropium
C. Sulbutamol
D. Sodium chromoglycerate

1413. Regarding theophylline, all are correct except :
A. Increased diaphragmatic contractilitis
B. Increased cardiac output
C. Suitable for nocturnal doses only
D. Increases antiproteaase activity

1414. Malignancy presenting as solitary pulmonary nodule is :
A. Melanoma
B. Breast carcinoma
C. Colon carcinoma
D. All of the above

1415. A.B.G. picture of early stage of bronchial asthma is :
A. Normal PaO2 PaCO2
B. Decreased PaO2 & increased PaO2
C. Decreased PaO2 & decreased PCO2
D. Decreased PaO2 & normal PCO2

1416. Most pulmonary thromboembolic originate from :
A. Deep vens of Calf
B. Deep veins of thigh
C. Pelvic veins
D. Inferior vena cava

1417. Highest incidence of postoperative pulmonary thromboembolism is seen with :
A. C.A.B.G
B. Hernia repair
C. Hip arthroplasty
D. Vagatomy

1418. Commonest bronchogenic carcinoma to caustate is :
A. Squamons cell
B. Small cell
C. Large cell
D. Adenocarcinoma

Ans.						
	1407. D	1408. A	1409. D	1410. A	1411. B	1412. D
	1413. D	1414. D	1415. C	1416. B	1417. C	1418. A

1419. Sarcoidosis showed be treated with steroids in all except :
A. Reticulonodular shadows on C x R
B. Hypercalcaemia
C. Uveitis
D. Elevated A.C.E.

1420. Activity of sarcoidosis in assessed by :
A. Serum calcium
B. Serum A.C.E levels
C. Gallium scanning
D. All of the above

1421. Features seen iwth bronchial asthma are all except :
A. Raised residual volume
B. Reduced vital capacity
C. Increased DLCO
D. Increased PaCO2

1422. Best indicator of adequate ventilation is :
A. Arterial PO2
B. Arterial PCO2
C. Minute ventilation
D. Dead space/Tidal volume (Vd/Vr)

1423. FIO2 delivered by month to mouth ventilation is :
A. 0.17
B. 0.20
C. 0.24
D. 0.28

1424. Swan Ganz Catheter can measure :
A. Mean arterial pressure
B. Left ventricular preload
C. Cardiac output
D. Lung compliance

1425. Bull's eye lesion on X-ray chest is found in :
A. Malignant melanoma
B. Ca thyroid
C. Choriocarcinoma
D. Renal carcinoma

1426. Commonest side effect of inhaled steroids is :
A. Adrenal supression
B. Hyderadrenal cortiasm
C. Oropharyngeal candidiasis
D. Immunosuppression

1427. β_2 stimulant with the maximum cardio stimulant activity is :
A. Sulbutamol
B. Perbutaline
C. Meloproterenol
D. Fenoterol

1428. Dose of theophylline should be reduced in all except :
A. CCF
B. Cor pulmonale
C. Renal failure
D. Hepatic failure

1429. Diagnostic criterion of A.B.P.A include all except :
A. Asthma
B. Pulmonary infreterates
C. Peripheral bronchiectasis
D. Eosinophila

1430. All are seen in emphysema except :
A. Reduced FEV1/FVC
B. Increased TLC
C. Increased Residual volume
D. Restrictive flow volume loop

Ans.						
	1419. D	1420. D	1421. D	1422. B	1423. A	1424. C
	1425. A	1426. A	1427. B	1428. C	1429. C	1430. D

1431. Bronchiectasis can be seen in :
A. Young syndrome B. IgA deficiency
C. Mounier-Kuhn syndrome D. None of the above

1432. Best test to diagnose deep venous thrombosis is :
A. Doppler ultrasound B. Impedence plethysmography
C. Ascending contrest renography D. Radio Nuclide scan

1433. Commonest ECG change of pulmonary thromboembolism is :
A. Sinus tachycardia B. Right axis deviation
C. Tall P waves D. ST changes

1434. Commonest X-ray finding in pulmonary embolism is :
A. Normal CxR
B. Elevated hemidiaphragm
C. Increased transluscency
D. Pulmonary infarct

1435. Commonest lung cancer in non smokers is :
A. Squamous cell B. Adenocarcinoma
C. Small cell carcinoma D. Large cell carcinoma

1436. Incorrect statement about small cell carcinoma is :
A. Ectopic hormone production
B. Responsive to chemotherapy
C. Central location
D. Associated hypercalcaemia

1437. Pneumonectomy can be done if FEV1 is greater than :
A. 1.0 Litre B. 1.5 Litre
C. 2.0 Litre D. 2.5 Litre

1438. Lung cancer most response to chemotherapy is :
A. Squamouns cell B. Adenocarcinoma
C. Small cell D. Large cell

1439. Hemothorax has a hemoatocrisis more than :
A. 10% B. 15%
C. 20% D. 25%

1440. Commonest cause of secondary pneumothorax is :
A. Asthma B. COPD
C. Tuberculosis D. Lung abscess

Ans.	1431. A	1432. C	1433. A	1434. A	1435. B	1436. D
	1437. A	1438. C	1439. D	1440. B		